André Luiz Silva Davim
Tereza Neuma de C. Dantas
Marcia R. Pereira

Bullfrog oil and its anti-inflammatory potential

AF376480

André Luiz Silva Davim
Tereza Neuma de C. Dantas
Marcia R. Pereira

Bullfrog oil and its anti-inflammatory potential

Anti-inflammatory potential of pure and microemulsified bullfrog oil

ScienciaScripts

Imprint

Any brand names and product names mentioned in this book are subject to trademark, brand or patent protection and are trademarks or registered trademarks of their respective holders. The use of brand names, product names, common names, trade names, product descriptions etc. even without a particular marking in this work is in no way to be construed to mean that such names may be regarded as unrestricted in respect of trademark and brand protection legislation and could thus be used by anyone.

Cover image: www.ingimage.com

This book is a translation from the original published under ISBN 978-613-9-63718-8.

Publisher:
Sciencia Scripts
is a trademark of
Dodo Books Indian Ocean Ltd. and OmniScriptum S.R.L publishing group

120 High Road, East Finchley, London, N2 9ED, United Kingdom
Str. Armeneasca 28/1, office 1, Chisinau MD-2012, Republic of Moldova, Europe
Printed at: see last page
ISBN: 978-620-7-68879-1

Copyright © André Luiz Silva Davim, Tereza Neuma de C. Dantas, Marcia R. Pereira
Copyright © 2024 Dodo Books Indian Ocean Ltd. and OmniScriptum S.R.L publishing group

ABSTRACT: Currently, the cost of treating patients with inflammatory diseases that progress systemically, especially sepsis, is very high and represents the biggest cause of death in non-cardiac intensive care units worldwide. In Brazil, the incidence of patients with sepsis is increasingly frequent. Despite pharmacological, technological and surgical advances, mortality from sepsis and/or associated diseases remains high worldwide, which is why we are looking for easily accessible, low-cost therapeutic alternatives to curb the progress of this disease. Natural products have been playing an important role in the pharmaceutical industry, as some of these substances act beneficially on the human immune system. Recently, there has been growing research into the possible biological and therapeutic properties attributed to bullfrog oil, as it has been used indiscriminately by the population to treat various diseases such as bronchitis, asthma, lichen sclerosus, furunculosis, sebaceous cysts and to heal skin and mucous membranes. However, the possible consequences of excessive consumption of this oil are increased production of eicosanoids derived from pro-inflammatory arachidonic acid and impaired liver regulation, predisposing to steatosis which can progress to liver inflammation and fibrosis. Many hypotheses are based on the action of the compounds present in bullfrog oil in modulating the inflammatory response, thus preventing the onset of tissue damage. In this way, microemulsion is a possible alternative for a new drug delivery system, with the aim of reducing the incidence of hepatoxicity and protecting the body against the onset of tissue damage as a result of the septic condition. The aim of this study was to evaluate the anti-inflammatory potential of pure bullfrog oil and a microemulsified system in an experimental model. In this study, a microemulsion system (WIV) was prepared and characterised and applied in biological tests in order to assess the anti-inflammatory potential of the pure oil and the microemulsion. The sepsis model, induced by the cecal ligant puncture (CLP) technique, and muscle damage induced by formalin were used. The tests were carried out on murine models, in which the animals were randomly separated into groups and treated with pure bullfrog oil and in microemulsion, using the gavage technique for subsequent evaluation of the hepatotoxic and anti-inflammatory potential. In order to analyse the anti-inflammatory potential in a sepsis model, bronchoalveolar lavages were carried out with subsequent counting of inflammatory cells and histopathological analyses of lung tissue. For the analysis of the muscle injury model, the horizontal extension of the animals' paws was assessed, as well as a histopathological analysis of the muscle tissue. To analyse the hepatotoxic potential of the substances, the survival rate of the animals after sepsis and histopathological analyses of the animals' liver tissues were assessed. When assessing the toxicity of pure bullfrog oil and the microemulsion system, it was observed that in the group administered the microemulsion (ME), the liver architecture was preserved, but with clinical signs of hepatic steatosis, unlike the pure bullfrog oil (OR) group, which showed multiple foci of hepatocytic necrosis accompanied by polymorphonuclear infiltrates. These findings indicate steatohepatitis, i.e. a more advanced stage and a precursor to hepatic carcinoma. When the survival of the animals was assessed, it was observed that the ME group had a significantly higher survival rate when compared to the OR group. When the anti-inflammatory potential of ME and OR was assessed in a sepsis model, the potential to modulate the inflammatory response was observed in both groups, given their ability to significantly (P< 0.01) reduce the migration of leukocytes to the lungs after sepsis induction. When the histology of the lung tissues of the animals from both groups was analysed, intense wear was seen in the animals from the OR group when compared to the ME group, where little tissue impairment was seen. In the muscle injury test, it was observed that the ME and OR groups showed good anti-oedematogenic potential up to the second hour of injury induction, when compared to the control group (P< 0.01), but no significant differences were observed between the two groups up to the twenty-fourth hour post-injury. Histological analyses showed greater wear and tear in the muscle tissue of the OR group, with intense presence of cellular infiltrate (oedema) and muscle fibre involvement, while the same intensity of injury was not observed in the ME group. Thus, it can be concluded

1

that pure bullfrog oil and oil in a microemulsion system have good anti-inflammatory potential in the models evaluated, although the pure oil showed high hepatotoxic potential, characterising it as a possible new drug delivery system (NSLF) in a microemulsion system.

Keywords: bullfrog oil; microemulsion system; sepsis; inflammation; toxicity.

Summary

CHAPTER 1

INTRODUCTION

Scientific reports suggest that natural products of various origins, whether plant or animal, have been playing an important role in different sectors of the industry, such as pharmaceuticals, because some of these substances act in a beneficial way on the human immune system. Many hypotheses are based on the action of these compounds in modulating the inflammatory response, thus preventing the onset of tissue damage.

Morbidity and mortality from sepsis is currently more common in intensive care units around the world, and has not been significantly reduced in recent decades.

Especially in Brazil, the incidence of patients with sepsis is increasingly frequent, but it is still difficult to determine the precise numbers due to the lack of notification, as well as due to cases that are associated with other severe illnesses. As a consequence of sepsis, many patients develop acute lung injury due to increased microvascular permeability. The lungs, being highly perfused organs, become possible targets for injury due to the excessive migration of immune system cells to the site of inflammation. Despite pharmacological, technological and surgical advances, mortality from sepsis and/or associated diseases remains high worldwide and the search for easily accessible, low-cost therapeutic alternatives is therefore important in an attempt to curb the progress of this disease.

Among the natural products with possible therapeutic potential are polyunsaturated fatty acids, but because their metabolism is hepatic, studies have shown their efficacy, although with serious restrictions due to the induction of hepatotoxicity. Frog oil, which is rich in polyunsaturated fatty acids, is a potential modulator of the inflammatory response and has therefore been used by various populations in Brazil for the treatment of numerous inflammatory diseases such as bronchitis, asthma, lichen sclerosus, furunculosis, sebaceous cysts and healing of the skin and mucous membranes. In an attempt to attenuate or even eliminate the deleterious effects of direct administration of polyunsaturated fatty acids, the use of microemulsion systems is a possible alternative as a drug release vehicle, since this system releases the fatty acids gradually, thus avoiding liver overload and consequently toxicity of this organ.

Microemulsions are considered efficient drug release systems and are characterised by being a mixture of two immiscible or partially miscible chemical substances, under the action of a surfactant that acts as an emulsifying agent, reducing interfacial tension and stabilising the solution. The microemulsion to be studied in this work is made up of bullfrog oil (BT), an aqueous solution and soya lecithin as a surfactant.

The aim of this study was to evaluate the anti-inflammatory potential of pure and microemulsified bullfrog oil in different experimental models.

To this end, the microemulsion tested in this study was prepared and characterised. Both the hepatotoxic potential and the survival rate of septic mice were analysed after treatment with pure bullfrog oil and the microemulsion. The levels of leukocyte migration to the lungs through bronchoalveolar lavage in septic mice and the histology of the lung parenchyma of these animals were also analysed. Finally, the anti-oedematogenic activity of pure and microemulsified bullfrog oil in a muscle injury model was analysed.

CHAPTER 2

THEORETICAL ASPECTS AND STATE OF THE ART

2.1 - MICROEMULSION SYSTEMS (SME)

Microemulsion systems used in drug formulation have the ability to modify the release rate of the compound, offering benefits that include increased solubility, absorption and control of the drug's bioavailability, reducing toxicity and increasing the compound's clinical efficacy (DAMASCENO et al., 2011). Thus, microemulsions (ME) function as reservoirs with the capacity to release active compounds into cells and can be applied without restriction by oral, ocular, parenteral, transdermal, vaginal and rectal routes of administration (GRUPTA et al., 2008; FIGUEIREDO et al., 2013).

Microemulsions (ME) are considered to be a new drug release system and their use in the pharmaceutical field is growing, since they have the ability to modify the speed of drug release, offering numerous benefits with good therapeutic safety.

Microemulsion systems (MES) were originally described by Hoar and Schulman in 1943. However, the term microemulsion was only used by Schulman in 1959 to define a transparent system obtained by titrating an emulsion with a medium-chain alcohol (DAMASCENO, 2011). After this, the use and application of these systems became widespread in the 1970s, with their use for advanced oil recovery during the energy crisis (NAJJAR, 2012).

Currently ME is described as a dispersion of an aqueous phase and an oily phase stabilised by a surfactant and/or a co-surfactant, where such a system is isotropically translucent, thermodynamically stable, single-phase, with low interfacial tension (USTUNDAG OKUR et al., 2011; PASCOA et al., 2015). The formulation of MEs can involve a combination of three to five components: oil, water, surfactant, co-surfactant and electrolyte. As well as being a thermodynamically stable system, another characteristic inherent to MEs is the small size of their droplets, which are in the order of 10 to 100 nm (SHAKEEL; RAMADAN, 2010; JADHAV et al., 2010). In addition, because it is an isotropically translucent system, the diameter is imperceptible to the naked eye and is less than % of the wavelength of the light, causing it to scatter little of the incident light (MUZAFFAR et al., 2013).

Taking into account the dispersed and dispersing phases, a ME can be classified as oil-in-water (O/W) when the spherical oil droplets are surrounded by surfactant molecules in a continuous water medium. Conversely, when spherical water droplets are surrounded by surfactant molecules in a continuous oil medium, this system is known as water-in-oil (W/O) (DAMASCENO, 2011). In addition to these two types of ME, there is the formation of a non-spherical structure with more structured configurations, known as bicontinuous (FANUN, 2009). Figure 1 shows an illustration of the three known types of EM.

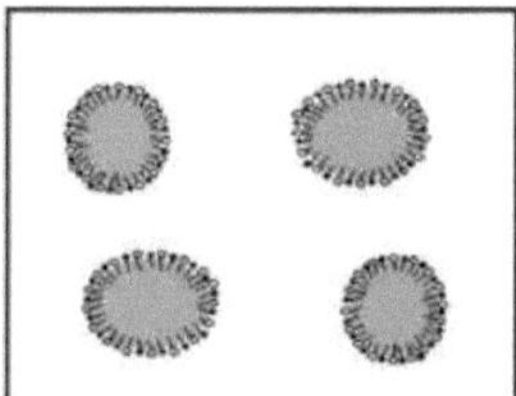
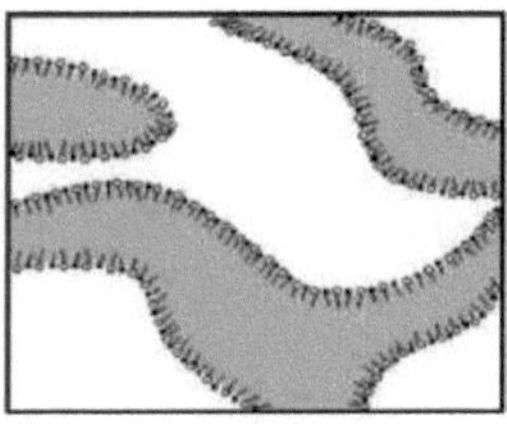
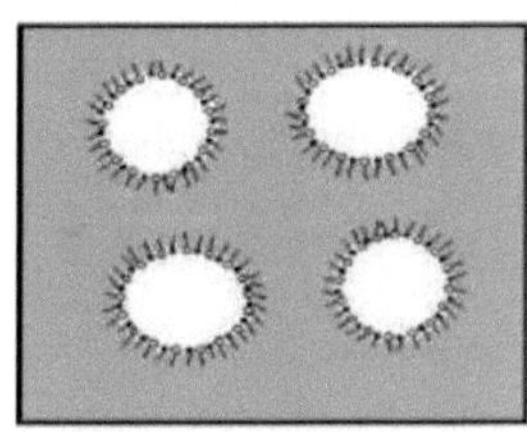

Figure 1: Types of microemulsions schematised by the oil phase (grey), the aqueous phase (white) and a surfactant/cotensoactive interfacial film.

(Source: Damasceno et al., 2011)

It is possible to establish differences between emulsion and microemulsion systems, ranging from particle size, appearance to the naked eye, stability, tension and the amount of surfactants, as shown in Table 1.

Table 1: Differences between emulsions and microemulsions

	EMULSION	MICROEMULSIONS
Size of dispersed droplets	1-10 μm	10-100 nm
Appearance	Cloudy and milky	Transparent and translucent
Stability	Thermodynamically unstable	Thermodynamically stable

| Interfacial tension | High | Very low |
| Quantity of surfactants | Low | High |

Source: Adapted from DAMASCENO, 2011.

The phase diagram is a tool used to describe the conditions under which microemulsions can be obtained and the transition boundary regions between emulsions and other systems. Ternary diagrams are considered to be graphical tools, as they allow data to be interpreted. The triangular diagram shows three associated variables - the aqueous phase, the oil phase and the surfactant, where each component takes up one of the vertices of the triangle (SILVA et al., 2009). Using ternary diagrams, it is possible to map the presence of different system equilibria, as classified by Winsor (1948): Winsor I (two-phase - shows microemulsion equilibrium with excess oil in the upper portion of the system); Winsor II (two-phase - shows emulsion equilibrium with excess water in the lower portion of the system); Winsor III (three-phase system - shows microemulsion equilibrium with excess oil and water); Winsor IV (homogeneous and single-phase system) (WINSOR,1948). Figure 2 shows a diagram containing the three phases, represented as A, B and C. Table 2 shows the characteristics of each phase according to Winsor's classification.

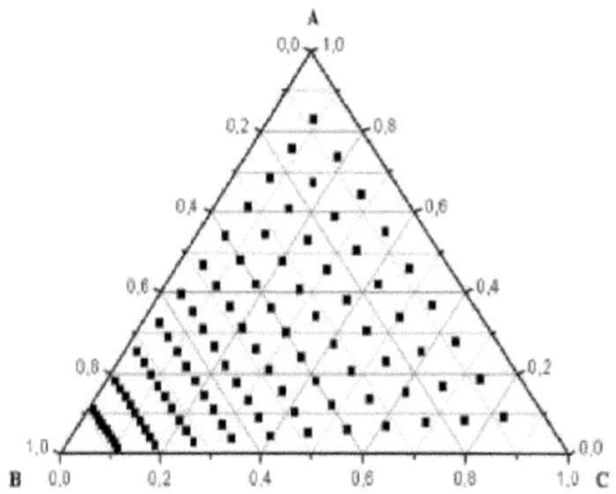

Figura 2: Representation of an equilateral triangle in which each component (aqueous phase, oil phase and surfactant) of the microemulsion assumes one of the vertices.

Source: DAMASCENO, 2011.

Winsor I	Winsor II	Winsor III	Winsor IV
Balance between emulsified phase and	Balance between the emulsified phase and	Equilibrium between	System with only the

8

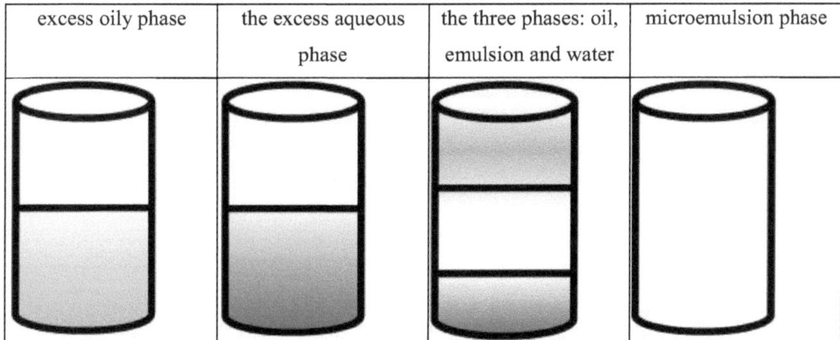

excess oily phase	the excess aqueous phase	the three phases: oil, emulsion and water	microemulsion phase

Figura 3:   It shows the microemulsion equilibria classified by Winsor. Aqueous phase: blue; oily phase: beige and emulsified phase: transparent.

Source: DAMASCENO, 2011.

With the advance of research, especially in the pharmaceutical field, into the treatment of various diseases using effective and viable chemical substances, there is growing concern about the adverse effects and potential toxicity caused by the use of these substances with pharmacological activities. Thus, recent studies describe modern and pharmacologically more efficient therapeutic alternatives, which present the possibility of reducing toxicity, increasing activity, therapeutic efficacy and bioavailability, as well as a controlled and targeted release of the active substance (BRUXEL et al., 2012; FIGUEIREDO at al., 2013).

Due to their peculiar characteristics, such as ease of preparation, thermodynamic stability, adequate viscosity, transparency and high capacity to solubilise drugs that are not very soluble in water in the oily disperse phase, the use of microemulsion systems has been considered as a therapeutic alternative, acting as a drug release system (DLS) (FIGUEIREDO et al., 2013).

2.2 - BULLFROG OIL

The bullfrog Rana (Lithobates) catesbeiana is an amphibian that is large in size compared to other amphibian species and has accelerated and continuous body growth throughout its life cycle (Figure 3), with high feeding and reproduction rates, territorial behaviour and generalist feeding habits.

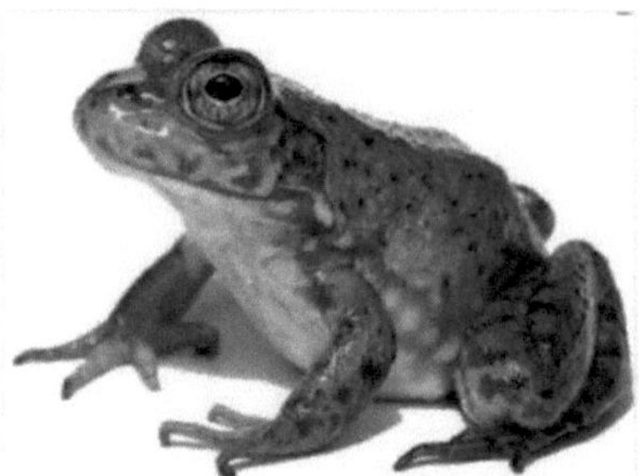

Figura 4: bullfrog of the species Rana catesbeiana

Source: www.biologycorner.com. Accessed on 16/05/2016.

The species Rana catesbeiana (also known as the bullfrog or giant bullfrog), taxonomically belongs to the Kingdom Metazoa, Phylum Chordata, Subphylum Craniata, Superclass Gnathostomata, Class Amphibia, Superorder Ranidae, Order Anura, Suborder Neobatrachia, Superfamily Ranonidae, Family Ranidae, Subfamily Raninae, Genus Rana, Subgenus Aquarana (BOELTER; CECHIN, 2007; FICETOLA, et al., 2007). The ranidae family has more than 9 genera and 300 identified species. The species in this family include smaller amphibians (Asians) and larger amphibians (Americans). After the eggs are laid and the tadpoles are released, they spend around 2 - 4 years in this form until they reach adulthood (ZUG, et al. 2001). The bullfrog lives preferentially in aquatic or humid environments (NÓBREGA, 2007). The species originated in the northern region of North America (PEREIRA, 2013), however, it has become an introduced species in many countries (Figure 4) due to the species' good adaptability and the high economic value attributed to it. The species was brought to Brazil in the 1930s and has been commercialised ever since, mainly by the food industry, with a significant expansion since the 1970s (CUNHA; DELARIVA, 2009).

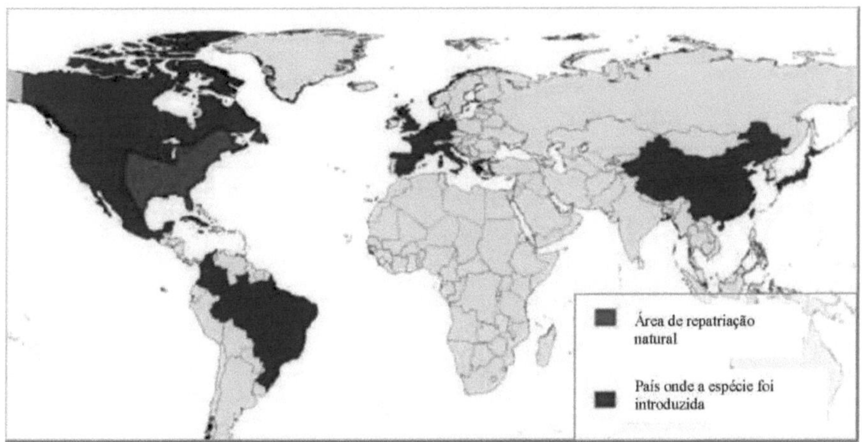

Figure 5: Geographical distribution of the bullfrog *(Rana catesbeiana)*
Source: www.adlayasanimals.wordpress.com - accessed on 20/05/2015.

The country's climatic conditions have favoured the development and reproduction of this type of amphibian, which is currently the most used species in Brazilian breeding facilities (Figure 5) (CUNHA; DELARIVA, 2009). The meat from the thighs of this species is widely commercialised; the carcass and legs are turned into feed for bullfrog tadpoles and the adipose tissue is used to extract oil. The by-products (skin, viscera and fat) are the object of scientific research aimed at their applicability in the pharmaceutical industry (LOPES et al., 2010). Brazil is currently one of the world's largest producers of the species *Rana catesbeiana*. The adaptive success of the bullfrog and the profitability proposals advocated by the practice of ranching have encouraged rural producers to invest in this activity, thus facilitating the spread of this species to various regions of the country (AGOSTINHO, 2003; CUNHA; DELARIVA, 2009).

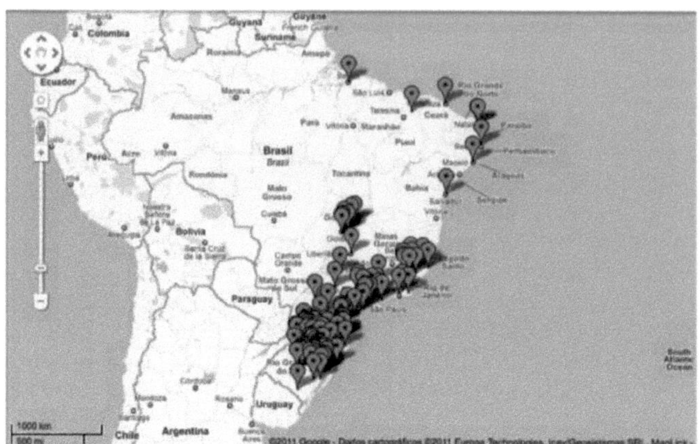

Figura 6: Geographical distribution of bullfrog breeding sites in Brazil
Source: www.ib.usp.br - accessed on 23/05/2015.

Bullfrog oil (BT) is extracted from the adipose tissue of the animal's abdomen, where the greatest amount of fat is concentrated, representing around 10 per cent of the amphibian's total weight. Currently, there is growing research into the possible therapeutic properties of OR, due to the presence of polyunsaturated fatty acids in its composition (LOPES, et al., 2010). Some studies have been carried out to assess the potential of OR in inflammatory processes (SILVA et al., 2004; PERINI et al., 2010), such as bronchitis, asthma, lichen sclerosus, furunculosis, sebaceous cysts and in the healing of skin (wounds) and mucous membranes (LOPES, 2007).

With regard to the levels of unsaturated fatty acids present in bullfrog oil, quality based on nutritional concepts consists of the presence of essential fatty acids, which are omega-3 and omega-6. According to MÉNDEZ et al. (1998), a total of 62 types of fatty acids have been identified, which have various effects on the immune and inflammatory response. Table 3 shows some of the fatty acids that have been identified in oils extracted from bullfrogs.

Table 3: Percentage of fatty acids present in oil extracted from bullfrog adipose tissue.

Fatty acid (%)	Chain	(Méndez, et al., 1998)	(Silva, et al., 2004)	(Lopes, et al., 2010)
Myristic acid	14:0	2,7	2,77	1,8

Palmitic	16:0	18,1	11,91	18,5
Stearic	18:0	4,1	2,34	3,2
Oleic	(18:1 n-9)	31,7	37,6	36,3
Linoleic	(18:2 n-6)	12,9	23,78	25,0
Linolenic	(18:3 n-3)	1,4	1,97	2,1
Palmitoleic	(16:1 n-7)	8,0	17,0	9,4
Eicosapentaenoic-EPA	(20:5 n-3)	1,5	0,46	-
Docosahexaenoic acid (DHA)	(22:6 n-3)	4,7	0,91	0,1
Arachidonic AA	(20:4 n-6)	-	0,74	0,6

According to Méndez et al. (1998) the main fatty acids found during the extraction of bullfrog oil were palmitic (18.1%), stearic (4.1%), myristic (2.7%), oleic (31.7%) and linoleic acid (12.9%); long-chain polyunsaturated fatty acids were also present in significant quantities, i.e. EPA (1.5%) and DHA (4.7%) (Table 3). These fatty acid concentrations were probably derived from the fishmeal content of the animal's diet, thus influencing the fatty acid concentrations.

According to Machado et al. (2016), in some studies that dealt with the chemical characterisation of bullfrog oil, the same compounds were identified for all the studies, but it was possible to find differences in the concentrations between the constituents. In this study by Machado, the concentration of arachidonic acid was 8.4%, while Silva, et al., (2004) and Lopes, et al., (2010), identified the same compounds with concentrations of 0.74% and 0.6%, respectively. There were significant differences in EPA (17.6%) and DHA (0.8%) compared to the studies by Silva, et al., (2004) (0.46% and 0.91%) and Lopes, et al., (2010) (0% to 0.1%) (Table 3). These differences may be related to both the diet of these amphibians and the climatic conditions of the ranches (MACHADO et al., 2016). The results obtained are relevant, considering that arachidonic acid acts as a pro-inflammatory agent, stimulating the synthesis of leukotrienes and prostaglandins, promoting the migration of leukocytes and accelerating the start of the first phase of the skin healing process.

Omega-3 has a suppressive effect as a producer of cytokines and antibodies, inhibition of lymphocyte proliferation, expression of adhesion molecules and activation of Natural Killer (NK) cells. Omega-6, on the other hand, has both inhibitory and stimulatory effects on the immune response (PERINI et al., 2010). Polyunsaturated fatty acids (PUFA) and the products derived from their cellular metabolism can modulate the activity of kinases involved in the activity of NF-kB (nuclear factor kappa B), which is an inflammation factor activated by the phosphorylation of the IkB protein. As a consequence of this activation, NF-kB migrates to the cell nucleus, binding to DNA sequences (kB sites) that are located in the promoter regions of genes related to apoptosis, cell adhesion, immune response, inflammation, cell stress and tissue remodelling. It is therefore believed that PUFAs may be important in the inflammatory process, as they are linked to the suppression of factors such as NF-kB, modulating its activity and reducing tissue wear due to the release of cytokines (POLETTO, 2011). Arachidonic acid (AA), a long-chain polyunsaturated fatty acid with 20 carbons, is formed from the linoleic acid (omega-6) present in the diet. AA metabolites (also called eicosanoids) influence a range of biological processes, such as inflammation and haemostasis, and have the ability to act as mediators in practically all stages of inflammation. In inflammatory responses, both their synthesis and inhibition interfere with inflammation. In the body, AA is a component of cell membrane phospholipids and is released through the activation of cellular phospholipases, which can be stimulated by inflammatory mediators such as C5a. Two enzymatic pathways are responsible for AA metabolism (Chart 1): cyclooxygenase, which stimulates the synthesis of prostraglandins and thromboxanes; and lipooxygenase, responsible for the production of leukotrienes and lipoxins.

Table 1 - Enzymatic pathways of arachidonic acid metabolism, their products and effects.

Via	Products	Effects
Cyclooxygenase	Prostraglandin	Vasodilation; Inhibition of platelet aggregation.
	Thromboxanes	Vasoconstriction; Promotion of platelet aggregation.
Lipooxygenase	Leukotrienes	Vasoconstriction;

| | Bronchospasm; Increased vascular permeability. |
| Lipoxins | Inhibition of neutrophil adhesion and chemotaxis. |

Adapted from the book: Fundamentals of Pathology. 7ª . edition

As you can see, AA plays an important role in the inflammatory process, since its metabolism produces various inflammatory mediators that will act in different ways in the body.

2.3 - BIOLOGICAL IMPORTANCE OF FATTY ACIDS

Fatty acids are carboxylic acids that make up one of the fundamental units of lipids. They are classified according to the number of atoms in the carbon chain - short, medium or long; as to the number of double bonds - saturated, monounsaturated and polyunsaturated and; as to the position of the first double bond - from its methyl radical, represented by the Greek letter omega (ω) or from its functional group, represented by the letter delta (Δ) (CASANOVA; MEDEIROS, 2011). Polyunsaturated fatty acids (PUFA) are so called because they contain two or more unsaturations and are characterised by the location of the double bonds. There are three important families of polyunsaturated fatty acids to consider: oleic acid (ω-9); linoleic acid (ω-6); and alpha linolenic acid (ω-3). Among them, those belonging to the omega-6 family stand out: linoleic acid (LA) and arachidonic acid (AA) and the omega-3 family: alpha-linolenic acid (ALA), eicosapentanoic acid (EPA) and docosahexaenoic acid (DHA) (PERINI et al., 2010).

Currently, there is growing interest in the role of polyunsaturated fatty acids on the inflammatory response and the immune system (SCORLETTI E.; BYRNE C. D., 2013). Bullfrog oil is rich in essential polyunsaturated fatty acids, omega-3 (ALA - alpha-linolenic acid) and omega-6 (LA - linoleic acid), which make up a class of molecules that are not synthesised by our bodies and must be supplied through the diet, They are found, respectively, in high concentrations in fish oils and in marine fish from cold and deep waters (mainly mackerel, sardines, salmon and trout) and in the seeds of oil-bearing plants (soya, corn and sunflower oils and nuts) (CASANOVA; MEDEIROS, 2011).

The biological functions of PUFAs are diverse, they play an important role in the structure of the cell membrane, in metabolic processes and in the production of eicosanoids - inflammatory mediators of lipid origin, interfering in various stages of the inflammatory response such as vascular contraction, chemotaxis, adhesion, diapedesis, cell activation and death, and also form the phospholipid layer of biological membranes, providing the normal functioning of membrane-associated complexes of enzymes and transmembrane transporters and regulating gene transcription, They also form the phospholipid layer of biological membranes, which provide the normal functioning of membrane-associated complexes of enzymes and transmembrane transporters and regulate gene transcription, generating an effect on the level of metabolic processes, controlling the level of lipid and carbohydrate metabolism in the liver. Most of these events occur through metabolites derived from arachidonic acid such as prostaglandins, leukotrienes, thromboxanes and lipoxins (PERINI et al., 2010; MAKSYMCHUK, 2014; NASCIUTTI et al., 2015).

One of the important and main functions of essential fatty acids is related to their enzymatic conversion into eicosanoids. These molecules are metabolites responsible for modulating the body's inflammatory response and include prostaglandins, prostacyclins, thromboxanes, leukotrienes and derivatives of hydroxylated fatty acids which, according to Casanova and Medeiros (2011), participate in various physiological and pathological processes and are potent regulators of cellular function. Eicosanoids are formed from the oxidation of arachidonic, di- homogamalinolenic (DHGL) and EPA acids through metabolisation pathways, which are: cyclooxygenase (COX, with COX-1 and COX-2 isoforms), lipoxygenase (LOX) and cytochrome P450 (CYP) or through non-enzymatic pathways. When the cyclooxygenase pathway is activated, important biological mediators are formed: prostaglandins - PGs with the PGE subtype, thromboxanes - TXs, with the TXA and TXB subtypes and prostacyclins (PCI), while the lipoxygenase pathway leads to the synthesis of leukotrienes - LTs with the LTA, LTB,

LTC, LTD and LTE subtypes (CASANOVA; MEDEIROS, 2011; DENNIS, E. A. & NORRIS, P. C., 2015). COX-1 and COX-2, although similar in their protein structure, are enzymes encoded by different genes. COX-1 is expressed constantly in most tissues (blood vessels, platelets, stomach, intestine, kidneys), and is therefore called a constitutive enzyme, and is also essential for maintaining the normal physiological state of these tissues, including control of renal blood flow, homeostasis, autoimmune responses, lung function and central nervous system, cardiovascular and reproductive functions. COX-2 is present at sites of inflammation and is expressed primarily by cells involved in the inflammatory process, such as macrophages and monocytes, and is induced by cytokines (IL-1, IL-2 and TNF) and other mediators at sites of inflammation (growth factors and endotoxins). For this reason, it is called an inductive enzyme (HILÁRIO et al., 2006).

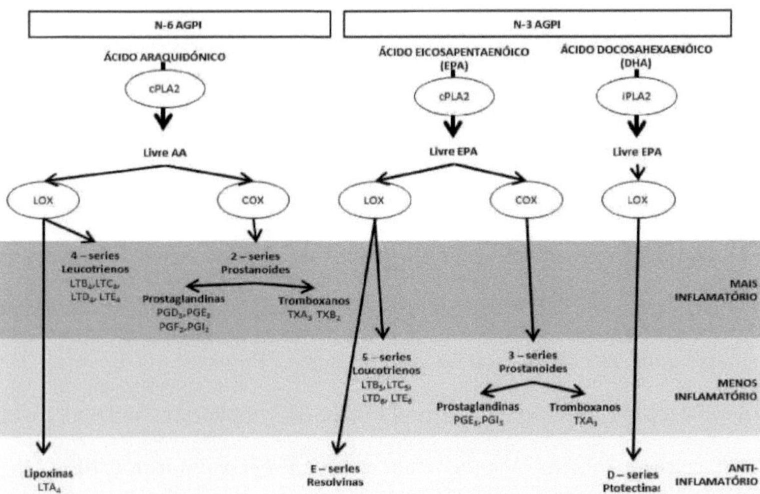

Figura 7:   Formation of eicosanoids derived from polyunsaturated fatty acids according to inflammatory state

(Source: Adapted from JOANNE et al., 2015)

Eicosanoids are metabolites considered to be an essential component of the innate immune response, as well as being part of a bioactive signalling network related to anti- and pro-inflammatory functions, regulating a diverse set of homeostatic and inflammatory processes related to various diseases. In addition, they play an important role in cell growth and differentiation, and act in the modulation of inflammatory and immune responses, since these metabolites are involved in modulating the intensity and duration of the inflammatory response and in regulating B and T lymphocytes (NASCIUTTI et al., 2015; DENNIS, E. A.; NORRIS, P. C., 2015). Studies involving eicosanoids in the inflammatory response mainly describe the signalling pathways activated by lipids produced through the COX enzyme,

since it has the ability to trigger signs of inflammation, including heat, swelling, redness, pain and loss of function. On the other hand, the signalling pathways activated by the LOX enzyme act more specifically during inflammation by promoting the recruitment of leukocytes to the sites of damaged tissue.The CYP pathways comprise a large number of enzymes that contain the heme iron and many CYPs are expressed in the liver (DENNIS, E. A.; NORRIS, P. C., 2015). Eicosanoids derived from omega-3 fatty acids have anti-inflammatory characteristics, while those from omega-6 fatty acids have proinflammatory characteristics when in excess in the body. Studies show that omega-6 fatty acids are precursors to the synthesis of eicosanoids of the par series, with proinflammatory characteristics, such as thromboxanes A2, protaglandins I2 and E2 (PGE2) and leukotrienes B4 (LTB4), which are highly active mediators in inflammation. PGE2 has various proinflammatory effects, including inducing fever, increasing vascular permeability and vasodilation, pain and oedema. However, PGE2 also has immunosuppressive effects, in that it reduces the proliferation of lymphocytes and the activity of Natural Killer (NK) cells and inhibits the production of tumour necrosis factor (TNF-α), IL1, IL2, IL6 and IFN-γ While LTB4 has proinflammatory characteristics, as it induces the release of lysosomal enzymes, increases the production of reactive oxygen species and TNF-α, IL-1 and IL-6 and increases vascular permeability. On the other hand, consumption of omega-3 fatty acids favours the synthesis of odd-series eicosanoids such as PGE3, TXA3 and LTB5, which have anti-inflammatory characteristics (PESCE et al., 2014).Thus, once ingested and absorbed, alpha-linolenic (ALA) and linoleic (LA) acids can be oxidised for energy production via 0-

oxidation, stored as energy (triglycerides, for example), deposited in structural components of a cell (phospholipids) or undergo a series of desaturation and elongation processes of the carbon chain to produce eicosanoids (Figure 7), processes that take place in the endoplasmic reticulum, especially in the liver (PERINI et al., 2010; NASCIUTTI et al., 2015). Linoleic acid (LA) can be elongated and desaturated to produce arachidonic acid (AA), which can then be metabolised by the cyclooxygenase (COX), lipoxygenase (LOX) and cytochrome P450 (CYP) pathways. AA is the precursor of series 2 protanoids (PGE2, TXA2, PCI2) and series 4 leukotrienes, which are considered proinflammatory because they have chemotactic, vasoconstrictive and platelet aggregating actions (CASANOVA; MEDEIROS, 2010; MONTEIRO et al., 2014), Similarly, alpha linolenic acid (ALA) can be elongated and desaturated to produce two long-chain fatty acids: eicosapentaenoic (EPA) and docosahexaenoic (DHA). EPA can also be metabolised by cyclooxygenase and lipoxygenase to form eicosanoids - series 3 prostanoids (PGE3, TXA3, PCI3) and series 5 leukotrienes, which are less proinflammatory than those derived from arachidonic acid. EPA and DHA can be metabolised into new anti-inflammatory compounds known as docosanoids (MONTEIRO et al., 2014).

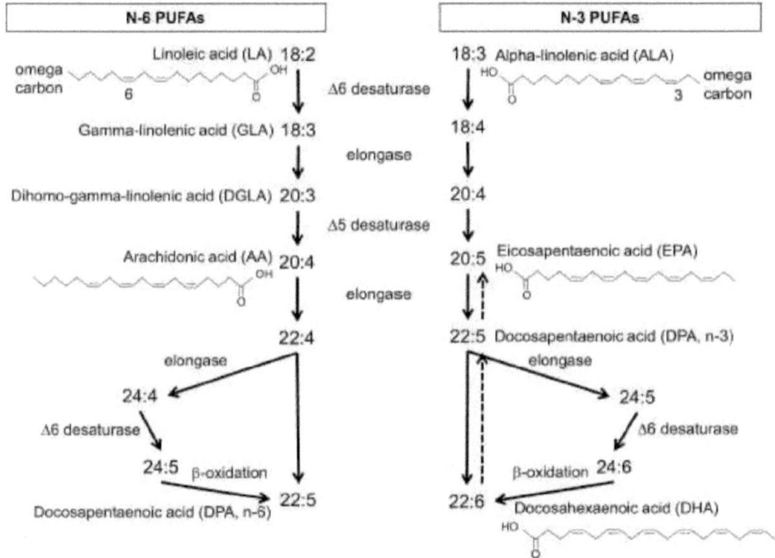

Figura 8: Metabolism of polyunsaturated fatty acids from the N3 and N6 family.

(Source: Adapted from JOANNE et al., 2015)

Studies show that EPA and DHA activate PPARα *{Peooxisome proliferator activated receptor} - a* marker of fatty acid oxidation, and inhibit SREBP *(Sterol regulatory element binding protein) - a* marker of fatty acid synthesis. EPA is the strongest PPAR activator and DHA is the most potent fatty acid regulator of SREPB (HANKE et al., 2013). PPARs are transcription factors from a family of nuclear receptors, characterised by their distribution pattern in tissues and their metabolic function, playing an important role in lipid and lipoprotein metabolism and in controlling the expression of fatty acid transporter and translocator proteins in cells, as well as participating in the control of the inflammatory process. PPARα participates in the control of inflammatory processes, since its activation prevents the transcriptional activity of NF-kB, which is the transcription factor responsible for the expression of cytokines and proinflammatory mediators, such as interleukin (IL) 6 and prostaglandins. Peroxisome proliferation is a cellular response to various situations, such as some pathophysiological conditions that involve drastic changes in cell morphology and peroxisome enzymatic activities. Nutritional factors such as diets rich in fats, especially those enriched with fish oils, induce peroxisome proliferation (CURI et al., 2002).

According to Nasciutti et al. (2015), studies show that diets with adequate amounts of omega-3 and omega-6 polyunsaturated fatty acids play important roles in the prevention of chronic inflammatory diseases, have an anti-inflammatory action and participate in immunomodulatory functions. This was first observed in an epidemiological study involving the Eskimo population, who are high consumers of EPA and DHA and showed a low incidence of inflammatory diseases, asthma, psoriasis and autoimmune diseases (CURI et al., 2002; MARTINS et al., 2008). Omega-3 fatty acids have suppressive effects such as the production of antibodies and cytokines, inhibition of lymphocyte proliferation, expression of adhesion molecules and activation of Natural Killer (NK) cells, which represent an important line of non-specific defence that recognises and lyses cells infected by viruses, bacteria, protozoa and also tumour cells, as well as recruiting neutrophils, macrophages and activating dendritic cells and T and B lymphocytes (PERINI et al., 2010; NASCIUTTI et al., 2015) and also has the ability to reduce serum triglycerides, promoting β-oxidation of fatty acids while inhibiting fatty acid synthesis in the liver (MONTEIRO et al. 2014). In contrast, omega-6 fatty acids have both inhibitory and stimulatory effects on the immune response (PERINI et al., 2010; NASCIUTTI et al., 2015).

In this way, the consumption and distribution of essential fatty acids in the plasma directly influences the properties that regulate the functions of cytokine release, eicosanoid formation, receptor function and cell membrane composition, and is also important in determining the severity of the inflammatory process (PERINI et al., 2010). Thus, the balanced proportion of omega-3 and omega-6 fatty acids in the diet plays an essential role in multiple biological processes, maintains metabolic homeostasis, and is of fundamental importance in controlling the inflammatory response, since the roles played by these acids in inflammation are antagonistic, while omega-3 is anti-inflammatory, omega-6 is proinflammatory (ELLULU et al. 2015; SZOSTAK et al., 2016).

2.4- EXCESS CONSUMPTION OF FATTY ACIDS POLYUNSATURATED

The essential fatty acids found in bullfrog oil have important functions such as maintaining cell membranes in normal conditions, brain functions, participating in the transfer of atmospheric oxygen to blood plasma, as well as having effects on the immune system and the inflammatory process. Due to the functions and benefits derived from the constituents of bullfrog oil, its consumption is growing in order to combat and treat various inflammatory diseases. However, its consumption should be moderate, since excess fatty acids can cause serious damage to the liver - hepatotoxicity, the organ responsible for metabolising these structures (SCORLETTI et al., 2013).

The liver plays a central role in lipid metabolism, as well as in the production and export of lipoproteins. In hepatocytes, free fatty acids can be metabolised through β-oxidation to generate ATP or esterified to produce triglycerides which are stored in lipid droplets within hepatocytes or packaged and released into the blood as very low density lipoprotein particles. Free fatty acids are derived from three different sources: dietary sources, de novo *lipogenesis* (DNL) from carbohydrates or amino acids and release from lipids stored in visceral adipose tissue or subcutaneous fat. Hepatic fat, which comes from the lipolysis of adipose tissue or the hydrolysis of lipoproteins, represents a ratio of 15% from dietary sources, 25% from DNL and 60% from free fatty acids (MILIÓ et aL, 2014).

Increased lipolysis of visceral adipose tissue results in the excess release of free fatty acids into the portal vein. When released into the portal circulation, the free fatty acids are then taken up by the hepatocytes mainly through the long-chain fatty acid synthase activity provided by members of the fatty acid transporter protein family. Once inside the hepatocyte, free fatty acids are bound to coenzyme A as fatty Acyl-CoA to form hepatic triglycerides, stimulate glucose-induced reduction in insulin uptake and induce intracellular inflammation. Thus, the accumulation of liver fat characterises hepatic steatosis and also contributes to the progression of non-alcoholic fatty liver disease - fibrosis, cirrhosis and hepatocellular carcinoma. The β-oxidation of fatty acids, which occurs in liver mitochondria, can be impaired by the increased load of free fatty acids in non-alcoholic fatty liver disease, resulting in the generation of reactive oxygen species. The result of oxidative stress leads to liver damage, inflammation and the initiation and progression of fibrosis (MILlC et al., 2014).

Excess consumption of fatty acids and reduced energy combustion are critical events that result in the storage of fat in the liver, causing fatty liver disease (FLD). Research shows that this disease is becoming a worldwide problem that affects the health of adults as well as children (MILIÔ et al., 2014), as a result of obesity, a sedentary lifestyle and a high-calorie, high-fat diet. When energy consumption exceeds energy combustion, the unburned energy is stored in the form of fat - triacylglycerol, in adipose tissue. Numerous complications can arise from excess fat storage, such as obesity, insulin resistance associated with obesity, diabetes mellitus, dyslipidaemia, hepatic steatosis, progressing to fatty liver disease (FLD) (LYONS et al, 2016).

Fatty liver disease (FLD) is classified clinically into two general entities: alcoholic FLD (AFLD) and non-alcoholic FLD (NAFLD). FLD has morphological characteristics consisting of hepatic steatosis, steatohepatitis, and can progress to the development of cirrhosis and hepatocellular carcinoma. NAFLD is the hepatic manifestation of metabolic syndrome, the incidence of which is increasing rapidly in adults and children (MILIC et al., 2014; THAN & NEWSOME, 2015). It is characterised by the excessive accumulation of low-density lipoproteins (VLDL) and serum triglycerides in the liver, and is critically influenced by host factors, including gender, age, the presence of diabetes, genetic polymorphisms and, more recently, the gut microbiota (THAN & NEWSOME, 2015). The manifestation of NAFLD can range from steatosis to non-alcoholic steatohepatitis (NASH), and can progress to cirrhosis, fibrosis and cellular hepatocarcinoma. NASH represents the inflammatory form that can lead to advanced fibrosis, cirrhosis and hepatocarcinoma and is defined histologically when 5% or more of the hepatocytes have intracellular triglyceride, in addition to lobular inflammation, microvesicular or macrovesicular steatosis (varying with the size of the lipid vacuoles) and hepatocellular degeneration in ballooning with or without Mallory bodies, in addition to portal or lobular inflammation, with or without fibrosis. (MAGALHÃES et al., 2014). It is also associated with an increased risk of developing cardiovascular disease, type 2 diabetes mellitus, insulin resistance, obesity, chronic kidney disease and colorectal cancer).

Excess free fatty acids and chronic inflammation derived from visceral adipose tissue (VAT) are considered two of the most important factors contributing to the progression of liver damage in NAFLD (*Non-alcoholic fatty liver disease*). In addition, secretion of adipokines from VAT as well as lipid accumulation in the liver promote further inflammation via nuclear factor kappa-B (NF-kB) signalling pathways, which are also activated by free fatty acids. In both the liver and visceral adipose tissue, hepatocytes and adipocytes are in close proximity to immune system cells *(Natural Killer - NK)*, hepatic stellate cells, Kupffer cells, endothelial cells and macrophages, with easy access to blood vessels and similar biochemical signalling pathways. In the liver, the inhibitor of nuclear factor kappa-B (IKK-β / NF-kB) is a signalling pathway activated by a high-fat diet, which is associated with the chronic inflammation that occurs in hepatic steatosis. In addition, it has been observed that hepatic production of the proinflammatory cytokines tumour necrosis factor (TNF-α), interleukin-6 (IL-6) and interleukin-iβ (IL-1β) is increased in animals subjected to a high-fat diet, indicating that lipid accumulation in the liver leads to subacute hepatic inflammation through NF-kB activation. Free fatty acids are capable of activating this pathway in the liver, increasing hepatic diacylglycerol (DAG) content, protein kinase-C (PKC) activity and plasma levels of MCP-1 (Monocyte Chemoattractant Protein-1). MCP-1 expression contributes to macrophage infiltration in adipose tissue and hepatic steatosis (MILIÓ et al., 2014).

Visceral adipose tissue (VAT) is a source of cytokines secreted by adipocytes, called adipokines. The best described adipokines are adiponectin, considered an insulin sensitiser, and leptin, a homone secreted mainly by adipocytes, which plays a functional role in the pathogenesis of non-alcoholic fatty liver disease (NAFLD). Leptin regulates energy intake and expenditure, metabolism and reproductive function, and also prevents the accumulation of lipids in non-adipose tissues such as the liver. Adiponectin acts by stimulating the secretion of anti-inflammatory cytokines such as interleukin-10 (IL-10) and inhibits the release of TNF-α and interleukin-6. In the liver, it acts through MAPK *(Mitogen Activated Protein Kinases),* PPAR-α (Peroxisome *proliferator-activated* receptor-$\alpha)$ and by inhibiting Toll-like receptor 4 (TLR-4) signalling. This cytokine is considered an element indicative of the severity of NAFLD (POLYZOS et al., 2011; SOUSA et al., 2015). Adipose tissue macrophages secrete high amounts of tumour necrosis factor (TNF-α) and interleukin IL-6, which suppress adiponectin production. The decrease in the circulating level of adiponectin in NAFLD is related to the amount of fat present in the liver. Thus, adiponectin acts by modulating the inflammatory response, as it increases fat oxidation by inactivating acetyl-CoA carboxylase, activating AMP-activated protein kinase and increasing the expression of the PPAR (Peroxisome proliferator activated *receptor*) gene (MILIC et al., 2014). TNF-α plays an important role in the progression of NAFLD to NASH and is produced by B lymphocytes, T lymphocytes (*Natural Killer*), macrophages and fibroblasts. It is a cytokine that has a lipogenic and fibrogenic effect, mediated by a paracrine mechanism that involves the activation of *Kupffer* cells with the secretion of soluble mediators that synthesise components of the extracellular matrix, and can even be used in the diagnosis of NAFLD/NASH (SOUSA et al., 2015).

Box 2: Role of different cytokines in NAFLD

Cytokine	Biological activity in experimental models	Biological activity in humans
Leptin	Proinflammatory stellate cell activation	Not elevated in NAFLD, no correlation with histology
Adiponectin	Anti-inflammatory	Lower in NAFLD than in controls; inverse relationship with fibrosis
TNF-α	Proinflammatory	High in NASH, correlates with fibrosis
IL-6	Uncertain	Studies in progress

Source: Adapted from Tsochatzis et al., 2009

Early diagnosis of fatty liver disease (FLD) is of the utmost importance, since 28% of patients who develop steatohepatitis can go on to develop cirrhosis and liver carcinoma, with a high risk of liver transplantation. Non-alcoholic fatty liver disease (NAFLD) is an emerging clinical-pathological condition characterised by the accumulation of lipids inside hepatocytes and is considered to be a syndrome of multifactorial aetiology, the most common factor being obesity. It presents various hepatic histopathological alterations, initially with hepatic fatty infiltration, which characterises hepatic steatosis, and can evolve with inflammatory activity and necrosis, with or without perisinusoidal fibrosis, which characterises steatohepatitis, advanced fibrosis and cirrhosis (MAGALHÃES et al., 2014). It is therefore one of the main causes of morbidity and mortality linked to liver disease. Studies show that, clinically, the majority of patients with NAFLD are asymptomatic, although some may present with fatigue, dyspepsia and hepatosplenomegaly, and have elevated liver marker enzymes *(aspartate aminotransferase - AST* and *alanine aminotransferase - ALT)* by approximately 20%. Studies show that free fatty acids generally circulate between the liver and peripheral adipocytes, without considerable accumulation of lipids in hepatocytes. There are two main pathways for the storage, mobilisation and metabolism of free fatty acids in the liver: triglyceride formation and subsequent release as very low density lipoproteins (VLDL) and mitochondrial P-oxidation to form acetyl-CoA. Research has shown that the onset of NAFLD is characterised by an increase in the intracellular content of triglycerides due to an imbalance between their synthesis and degradation, since the increased flow and/or endogenous synthesis of free fatty acids can lead to the accumulation of triglycerides in hepatocytes if mitochondrial β-oxidation and the production and secretion of VLDL are insufficient to cope with the load of free fatty acids. Lipid overload in hepatocytes can reach toxic levels, which generates an increase in oxidative stress with the formation of reactive oxygen species (free radicals), associated with mitochondrial damage, causing hepatocyte rupture or apoptosis and the release of triglycerides and toxic fatty acids, an event that stimulates the inflammatory response (MAGALHÃES et al., 2014).

Thus, the accumulation of lipids causes alterations in all phases of metabolism, resulting in excessive absorption of free fatty acids, accumulation of triglycerides, increased hepatic lipogenesis, decreased β-oxidation and secretion of VLDL; oxidative stress causes the release of various cytokines such as TNF-α, growth factor β and interleukins by Kupffer cells; reactive oxygen species activate stellate cells that participate in fibrinogenesis, and the products of lipid peroxidation and proteins modified by reactive oxygen species develop immunogenic properties causing the inflammatory response (MAGALHÃES et al., 2014).

Morphologically, hepatic steatosis manifests as an accumulation of large or small fat droplets in the cytoplasm of liver parenchyma cells, characterising macrovesicular and microvesicular steatosis, respectively. Studies show that in macrovesicular steatosis, hepatocytes contain a large fat vacuole that fills the cytoplasm and displaces the nuclei to the periphery, and can manifest in zone 3, predominantly with increasing severity. On the other hand, microvesicular steatosis occurs due to a genetic disorder and toxins, the hepatocytes are occupied by numerous small fat droplets that do not cause the nucleus to move to the periphery and tends to be more severe and progressive (REDDY et al., 2006; MAGALHÃES et al., 2014). Studies investigating the composition of hepatic fatty acids in patients with hepatic steatosis have revealed that the lipid profile of omega-3 polyunsaturated fatty acids is low, especially EPA and DHA. This suggests that omega-3 may play an important role in the treatment and prevention of hepatic steatosis, acting to increase hepatic fatty acid oxidation through the activation of PPAR and decrease fatty acid synthesis through SREBP, resulting in the regulation of genes involved in fatty acid synthesis (HANKE et al., 2013; MONTEIRO et al., 2014). Although polyunsaturated fatty acids belonging to the omega-3 family (EPA and DHA) have a potential anti-inflammatory effect, preventing the progression of simple hepatic steatosis to steatohepatitis and, consequently, preventing the development of NAFLD (Non-alcoholic fatty liver desease) (HANKE et al., 2013), excess consumption of these fatty acids, as well as those belonging to the omega-6 family, can cause serious damage to the liver, playing a fundamental role in the pathogenesis and progression of non-alcoholic fatty liver disease, which represents a spectrum of conditions related to fatty liver and originates with the accumulation of fat in the liver (hepatic steatosis), and can progress with the development of liver inflammation and fibrosis, to steatohepatitis (SCORLETTI et al., 2013).

CHAPTER 3

THEORETICAL BACKGROUND

3.1 - INFLAMMATION

The homeostasis of the human organism can be disrupted by aggressions of various kinds, where situations identified as abnormal or pathological trigger a set of defence mechanism reactions. Inflammation is a physiological process in which tissues rich in blood vessels respond to injury and a large number of mediators act to contain and/or eliminate the aggressors (ROBBINS et al., 2000). According to Abbas and Lichtman (2005), these agents can be microorganisms or parts of them, exogenous or endogenous foreign bodies, as well as agents that cause burns. The tissue damage caused by these agents initiates a series of molecular events, resulting in the production of pro-inflammatory mediators that promote the classic signs of inflammation.

However, the immunological response to inflammation is an important adaptive mechanism that allows the host to react, thus avoiding tissue damage. This reaction can be mediated by two fronts called humoral immunity and cellular immunity. When there is inflammation, there is an increase in the drainage of liquids and materials through the lymphatic vessels, which results in the displacement of these materials towards the regional lymph nodes rich in macrophages, Robbins (2000).

According to Pereira (1996) macrophages, like all the cells in the immune system, originate from undifferentiated cells in the bone marrow and, as well as exerting intense endocytic activity, secrete enzymes, plasma proteins, reactive oxygen species (ROS), prostaglandins and cytokines. In this way, macrophages play an important role in immune regulation and protection against infection. According to their state of activation, macrophages are classified as resident, inflammatory and activated. Resident macrophages are present in tissues and show functional activity and low ROS production.

When they are exposed to the lymphokines released by stimulated lymphocytes, they produce a high level of ROS, enabling them to destroy microorganisms. In addition, macrophages can destroy tumour cells by increasing their phagocytic activity. Macrophage activation is accompanied by increased oxygen consumption followed by unielectronic reduction, leading to the formation of ROS. The activation of these cells occurs when a foreign particle comes into contact with the plasma membrane, for example a bacterium, triggering the process through the activation of an enzyme complex associated with the plasma membrane.

In addition to the complement system, some mediators stand out, such as cytokines and pro-inflammatory peptides (MCGILL et al., 1998). According to Carvalho and Trotta (2003), with the release of these pro-inflammatory mediators, changes in cell adhesion properties are rapid and severe, causing an increase in adhesion between leukocytes and the endothelium. In this way, leukocytes are directed from the blood to the tissues by means of cell-to-cell signalling, involving initial contact with the vascular endothelium, a process mediated by specific adhesion molecules present on leukocytes and endothelial cells. Some of these molecules are integrins (mainly b1 and b2), intercellular adhesion molecules (ICAM-1, 2,3), vascular cell adhesion molecules (VCAM-1) and platelet-endothelium cell adhesion molecules (PECAM-1).

Among the leukocytes, neutrophils, also known as polymorphonuclear neutrophils (PMN), are the host's first line of defence against microorganisms and are recruited by diapedesis to inflammatory sites with the help of chemoattractant substances (FANTONI, 1999). Kotani (1999) emphasises that after migration, these leucocytes show phagocytic activity and also produce large quantities of ROS and reactive nitrogen species (RNS), such as hydrogen peroxide and nitric oxide, which are fundamental to the success of these cells' microbicidal action.

The recruitment of leukocytes to the site of inflammation involves a multi-step sequence of events, ranging from activation, rolling, adhesion to transmigration (diapedesis), coordinated by adhesion molecules expressed on the surface of leukocytes and endothelial cells that are involved in leukocyte-endothelium interaction. The initiation of neutrophil rolling is mediated by the reversible binding of selectins (glycoproteins) found on both the neutrophil surface (L-selectins) and the endothelium (E-selectin) (THOMAS et al., 2008). This recruitment to the tissues is extremely important in inflammation, but an exacerbated accumulation of these cells can lead to various problems and a variety of inflammatory diseases, such as meningitis, sepsis and systemic inflammatory response syndrome (SIRS). These inflammatory diseases, in turn, can induce tissue damage in organs that are highly vascularised, such as the lungs, nervous tissue, kidneys and organs of the gastrointestinal system, due to increased microvascular permeability (XIE et al, 2000; LAGAN et al., 2008). Figure 8 shows the migration of immune system cells to the site of inflammation, following signalling by inflammatory cytokines.

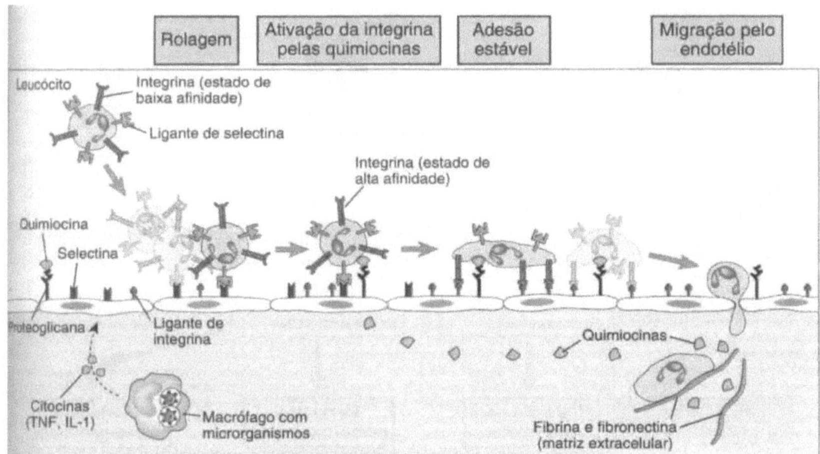

Figura 9: Neutrophil migration to the site of inflammation.

Pathology. Robbins & Cotran. 7ª Edition.

3.2 - SEPSE

3.2.1 - HISTORY

Pierre Adolphe Piorry (1794-1879), a French doctor, introduced the medical term septicemia (putrid blood poisoning) and pyaemia (pus in the blood) without establishing the differences and the pathogenic mechanisms involved (FERRAZ, 2008). Semmelweis, in the 19th century, was the first researcher to develop a modern view of sepsis. Lister, Halstead and Vong Bergmann, contemporaries of Semmelweis, also developed antisepsis techniques that resulted in a major reduction in the incidence of mortality caused by infections (MOUTA Jr., 2007). Clinical and experimental research throughout the 20th century led to a better distinction between the components of the pathophysiology of sepsis. In 1991, the Society of Critical Care Medicine and the American College of Chest Physicians were convened to standardise terminology related to the pathophysiology, severity of inflammatory conditions secondary to infection and sepsis therapy (BONE et al., 1992a; BONE et al., 1992b).

3.2.2 - CONCEPT

Sepsis *is* a term derived from the Greek verb "sepe/n", which means to putrefy or rot and more than 2700 years ago was a term used in Homer's poems (CATENACCI, KING, 2008; CHANG et al., 2010). Conceptually, sepsis is a pathology associated with inflammation, characterised as a complex syndrome arising from an uncontrolled systemic inflammatory response in the individual, of infectious origin, triggering multiple and decompensated organic manifestations with a high incidence of patient morbidity and mortality (KAO et al., 2007). Sepsis is a set of inflammatory, neural, hormonal and metabolic reactions known as the Systemic Inflammatory Response Syndrome (SIRS) resulting from a complex interaction between the infecting microorganism and the host's immune, pro-inflammatory and pro-coagulant response. SIRS is defined by the presence of at least two of the following clinical signs: temperature above 38°C or below 36°C, tachycardia with heart rate above 90 beats per minute, tachypnoea with respiratory rate above 20 respiratory movements per minute or hyperventilation with PaCO2 below 32 mmHg, leucocytosis above 12,000/mm³ , leucopenia below 4,000/mm³ or more than 10% of young neutrophil forms (sticks). The concurrence of two SIRS criteria with a presumed or obvious infectious focus confirms the diagnosis of sepsis. The association of sepsis with organ dysfunction and disturbed tissue perfusion characterises severe sepsis. The presence of sepsis-induced hypotension or persistent alterations in tissue perfusion after adequate haemodynamic resuscitation is called septic shock. In addition, multiple organ dysfunction syndrome is the presence of altered organ function in which homeostasis cannot be maintained without intervention (VIANA, 2011; DELLINGER et al., 2013). This syndrome is one of the most important infectious complications in contemporary medicine, both because of its incidence, its severity and its high potential for death (high lethality, depending on the stage at which the diagnosis is established) (SIQUEIRA-BATISTA et al., 2009; HOTCHKISS R.S.; KARL I.E., 2003). From a clinical point of view, the presentation of sepsis is related to the multiple possibilities of interaction between humans and microorganisms (SIQUEIRA-BATISTA et al., 2009), distinguishing situations such as infection, SIRS, sepsis, severe sepsis, septic shock and dysfunction of multiple organs and systems (AMERICAN, 1992; LEVY M. M. ET AL., 2003; PEREZ M. C. A., 2009). Table 2 describes the terms and concepts related to microorganisms, pathologies and physiological changes.

Chart 3: Definitions useful for understanding sepsis.

Term	Concept
Colonisation	This refers to the presence of microorganisms in a given location, without any damage being done to the host.
Infection	Presence of a certain agent that is causing damage to the host (inflammatory response to the microorganism is present).
Bacteraemia	Occurrence of viable bacteria in the blood, which can be transient; by extension, viremia, fungalemia and parasitem ia can be characterised.
Systemic inflammatory response syndrome (SIRS)	Characterised by being a non-specific response of the body to a variety of situations that generate inflammation - infection, burns, acute pancreatitis, trauma, and others. Two of the following conditions are required for its detection: Temperature > 38.0 °C or < 36.0 °C Heart rate > 90 bpm Respiratory rate > 20 irpm or PaCO, < 32 mmHg Leucocytes > 12,000/mm⁵ or < 4,000/mm- or > 10% bastons
Sepsis	SIRS triggered by a bacterial, viral, fungal or parasitic infection.
Hypotension	Systolic blood pressure < 90mmHg or a reduction of 40mmHg from "baseline" pressure.
Severe sepsis	Those associated with organ dysfunction, tissue hypoperfusion (characterised, among other things, by oliguria, acute mental disturbance and/or lactic acidosis) or arterial hypotension.
Septic shock	Hypotension (not attributable to another cause) with tissue hypoperfusion caused by sepsis. It can be *early*, when it lasts less than an hour (in response to infusion of crystalloid solution. 0.5-1 litre), or *late*, lasting more than an hour with or without the need for vasoactive amines.
Dysfunction of multiple organs and systems (DMOS)	Alterations in the function of the organs of a seriously ill person, so that homeostasis cannot be maintained without therapeutic intervention. *Primary* is the result of the injury itself (e.g. respiratory failure secondary to severe community-acquired pneumonia) and *secondary is* the result not of the injury, but of the host's organic response to the morbid condition (e.g. acute respiratory distress syndrome in a patient with acute necrotic pancreatitis).

Source: American, 1992; Levy M. M. et al., 2003; Perez M. C. A., 2009.

3.2.3 - IMMUNE RESPONSE AND PATHOPHYSIOLOGICAL ASPECTS.

The innate immune response is responsible for the initial inflammatory process in sepsis. It is mediated by pattern recognition receptors, such as Toll-like receptors (TLR) and CD14, which recognise pathogens or their products, identified as PAMPs (pathogen *associated molecular* patterns*)* (KORTEGEN A. et al., 2006; MEDZHITOV R.; JANEWAY JR. C.A., 1998). TLR-2 recognises peptide glycans from Gram-positive bacteria, while lipopolysaccharides (LPS) from Gram-negative bacteria are recognised by TLR-4 (COHEN J., 2002; RUSSEL J.A., 2006). LPS (Fig. 9) is a bacterial endotoxin present in the cell wall of Gram-negative bacteria, and is composed of a glycolipid complex, presenting a hydrophobic domain known as lipid A, which represents an invariable pattern comprising one of the most potent microbiological initiators of inflammatory processes (MILLER et al., 2005), 2005), where a short exposure to this agent is sufficient to activate monocytes and macrophages to synthesise and release pro-inflammatory cytokines such as IL-1, IL-6, IL-8 and IL-12. The production of these inflammatory mediators is extremely important for fighting pathogenic microorganisms; however, if produced in an uncontrolled manner, they can cause serious damage to the organism, such as microcirculatory dysfunction, tissue injury and septic shock (sepsis), which can result in the death of the host (FUJIHARA et al., 2003; COELHO et al., 2005).

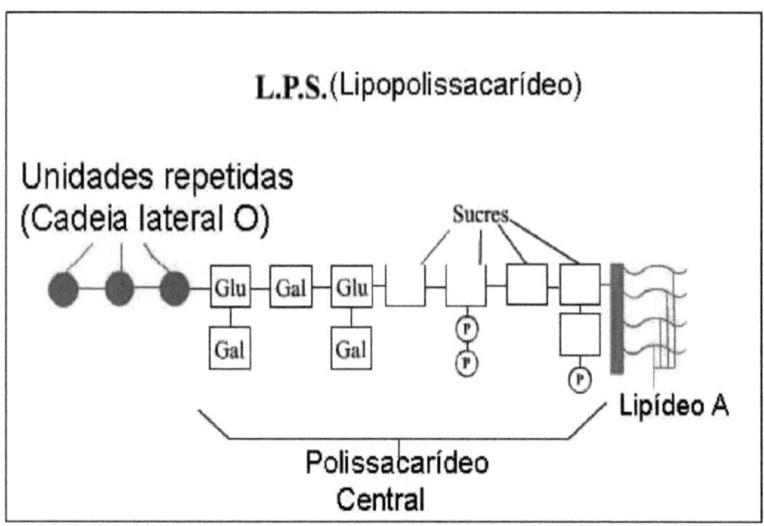

Figure 10: Schematic representation of the LPS molecule.
Source: Author

LPS recognition involves a complex of receptors in which the LPS-binding protein (LBP), CD14 and the mammalian Toll-like receptor (Toll-4/TLR4) act.

Enterobacterial LPS first interacts with LBP present in serum, causing a conformational change in this protein, which in turn transfers this LPS to the CD14 molecule present on the surface of monocytes and myeloid cells (HENKIN et al., 2009). Stimulation by LPS is followed by an increase in the physical proximity between CD14 and TLR4, which leads to TLR4 activation, thus generating biochemical signals through its intracytoplasmic tail, which trigger transcription factors that are responsible for stimulating the genes that encode the aforementioned pro-inflammatory cytokines (FUJIHARA et al., 2003; MILLER et al., 2005).

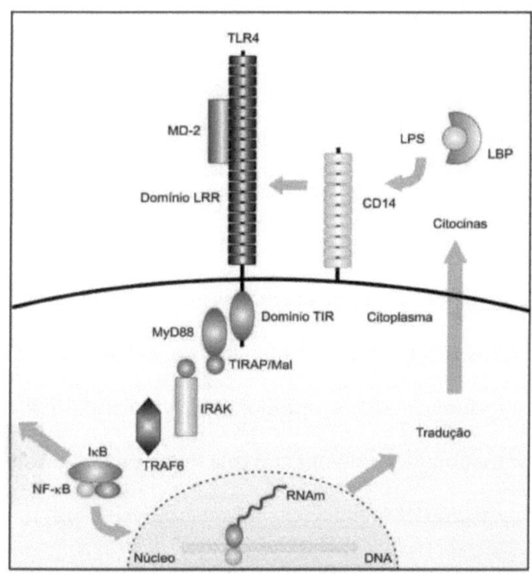

Figure 11: Molecular mechanism of gene activation and synthesis of pro-inflammatory cytokines.

Source: Author

Other cell surface molecules also recognise LPS: macrophage scavenger receptor (MRS), CD11b/CD18 and ion channels (HENKIN et al., 2009). Intracellular signalling depends on the binding of the cytoplasmic domain of the TLR, TIR (Toll-IL-1 receptor homology domain), to IRAK-4 (IL-1 receptor-associated kinase), a process facilitated by two adapter proteins, MyD88 (myeloid differentiation protein 88) and TIRAP (TIR domain-containing adapter protein) and inhibited by a third protein, Tollip (Toll-interaction protein). Cells can also respond to LPS via intracellular receptors known as NOD (nucleotide-binding oligomerisation domain) proteins. The mechanism by which the NOD recognises LPS in the cytosol is unknown (COHEN, 2002). Once activated, TLRs trigger a cascade of intracellular events that culminates in the nuclear translocation of NF-kB, a transcription factor that promotes the gene expression of pro-inflammatory molecules such as tumour necrosis factor alpha (TNF-α) and interleukin 1 beta (IL-1β) and also anti-inflammatory cytokines such as interleukin 10 (IL-10) (BALDWIN, 2001).

TNF-a and IL-1β activate the adaptive immune response, which is responsible for amplifying innate immunity. This is characterised by the activation of B cells which release immunoglobulins that facilitate the presentation of antigens to phagocytic cells (RUSSEL, 2006). In addition, T helper type 1 (Th1) cells promote positive feedback by secreting pro-inflammatory cytokines (TNF-α and IL-1β). Counterbalancing this mechanism, T helper type 2 (Th2) cells secrete anti-inflammatory interleukins (IL-4, IL- 10) (ABBAS et al., 1996). Pro-inflammatory cytokines increase the expression of adhesion molecules on leukocytes and endothelial cells. Although activated neutrophils destroy microorganisms, they also cause an increase in vascular permeability, leading to tissue oedema. In addition, activated endothelial cells release nitric oxide, a potent vasodilator that plays a fundamental role in the pathogenesis of septic shock (RUSSEL et al., 2006). The activation of monocytes and macrophages and the intense action of the initial mediators lead to the synthesis of other cytokines, such as IL-6, IL-8, IL-10 and HMGB1 (high mobility group protein box 1), with various synergistic and antagonistic effects on the inflammatory response. The secretion of IL-6 leads to the reprogramming of hepatic gene expression, the so-called "acute phase response", characterised by the production of acute phase proteins such as C-reactive protein and the suppression of negative acute phase proteins such as albumin (KORTEGEN et al., 2006). Excess production of LPS by Gram-negative bacteria can lead to sepsis, which is a devastating disorder characterised by intense production of pro-inflammatory cytokines and can lead to multiple organ failure and death (KARIMA et al., 1999).

3.2.4 - COAGULATION CASCADE

In addition to inflammation, microorganisms also activate the coagulation cascade, with an increase in pro-coagulant factors and a reduction in anticoagulant ones (RUSSEL, 2006; AIRD, 2003).The coagulation cascade is made up of a series of chain reactions, where once a serine protease is activated, it is available to activate all subsequent substrates. These reactions take place in activated phospholipid membranes and in some cases are accelerated by the presence of cofactors such as factor VIIIa and Va. For every pro-coagulant response there is a natural anticoagulant reaction (AIRD, 2003). Coagulation is initiated by the expression of tissue factor (TF) on the surface of endothelial cells and monocytes, an event that can be triggered by bacterial products such as endotoxins and cell surface components or by proinflammatory cytokines (MARSHALL J. C.; PANACEK E. A.).

LPS stimulates endothelial cells to produce tissue factor, which on the cell surface activates factor VII, resulting in the factor VIIa and tissue factor complex that converts factor X into Xa. Together with factor Va, factor Xa converts prothrombin into thrombin, which in turn results in the cleavage of fibrinogen into fibrin. Although the deposition of fibrin plays an important role in homeostasis and the localisation of microorganisms, intravascular coagulation prevents oxygen from reaching the tissues and can induce a new inflammatory lesion. In turn, the thrombin receptor activates NFκB, causing the transcription of inflammatory mediator genes and the synthesis of nitric oxide (MARSHALL J. C.; PANACEK E. A.). Endogenous anticoagulant factors such as protein C, protein S, antithrombin III and the Tissue Factor *Pathway Inhibitor* (TFPI) modulate coagulation, increasing fibrinolysis and removing microthrombi. In sepsis, LPS and TNF-α decrease thrombomodulin synthesis and the endothelial protein C receptor, preventing protein C activation and increasing plasminogen activator inhibitor 1 (PAI-1) synthesis, ultimately interrupting fibrinolysis (RUSSEL, 2006).

3.2.5 - CELL METABOLISM AND MECHANISMS OF ORGAN DYSFUNCTION

Sepsis causes changes in cellular metabolism that affect lipid, carbohydrate and protein metabolism. The inadequate supply of oxygen to the tissues as a result of the drop in blood flow in the capillaries and the reduction in cardiac output contributes to an increase in anaerobic metabolism and hyperlactataemia. However, even in the presence of an adequate oxygen supply, inefficient oxygen extraction and utilisation can occur at mitochondrial level (O'BRIEN et al., 2007), leading some researchers to speculate that there would be cellular hibernation, similar to that which occurs in myocardial ischaemia (HOTCHKISS R. S.; KARL I. E., 2003). One of the main consequences of mitochondrial dysfunction is a reduction in ATP production, which can persist even after the supply of substrates has been restored, a condition known as cytopathic hypoxia (HUBBARD et al., 2004).

The precise mechanisms that lead to organ dysfunction in sepsis have not been fully elucidated. Regardless of changes in the supply of oxygen and substrates, cells can react to septic aggression by modifying their behaviour, function and activity. The mechanisms responsible for organ dysfunction in sepsis can be grouped into systemic and organ-specific (ABRAHAM E.; SINGER M., 2007). Systemic mechanisms include alterations in vascular function and glucose metabolism. Vascular function is affected by a combination of numerous factors, such as hypovolaemia and vasoplegia. Among the factors involved in this process are: excessive production of nitric oxide, activation of potassium channels and changes in the levels of hormones such as cortisol and vasopressin. The acute toxicity caused by high levels of glycaemia can result in oxidative stress, with serious damage to mitochondrial function, particularly in cells where its utilisation is insulin-dependent. The organ-specific mechanisms are still poorly understood by the scientific community.

Why does an infection stimulate a systemic inflammatory response that affects some organs and not others? Some systems manage to escape relatively easily, while others are severely and prematurely compromised (ABRAHAM E.; SINGER M., 2007). The cardiovascular system is one of the most affected by the response that occurs in severe sepsis and septic shock. It has been known since the 1980s that in sepsis there is depression of myocardial function, even in patients with high cardiac output, with recovery in 7 to 10 days in those who survive. This myocardial dysfunction is the result of multiple cellular alterations, such as the effect of cytokines, nitric oxide, lysozymes 6 and C, bacterial DNA and RNA (RABAUEL C., 2006). The lungs are involved early on in the inflammatory process that occurs in sepsis. Acute lung injury is characterised by neutrophil activation, interstitial oedema, loss of pulmonary surfactant and fibrin-rich alveolar exudate. These alterations can be aggravated by an inadequate ventilation technique, at the expense of high airway pressures and oxygen toxicity. Post-mortem studies have shown that these changes are more pronounced on the epithelial side of the alveolar-capillary membrane, with apoptosis and cell necrosis being possible causes (ABRAHAM E.; SINGER M., 2007).

The brain is sensitive to the presence of microorganisms and inflammation through different mechanisms. Patients with sepsis may present with agitation, mental confusion or coma. In autopsy studies, various types of brain damage are found, such as ischaemia, haemorrhage or microabscesses. As the brain modulates its response through three afferent pathways - the hypothalamic-pituitary-adrenal axis, the sympathetic nervous system and the cholinergic anti-inflammatory pathway - it affects other organs and systems through neuroendocrine stimulation. The hepatosplanchnic system can be affected directly and, just like the brain and lungs, it can affect other systems at a distance. As the portal system drains directly into the liver, a third of the blood flow that circulates comes directly from the systemic circulation, which gives it a prominent role in identifying microorganisms or their products. The liver is also involved in the production of acute phase proteins. Clinical findings of liver dysfunction occur late in sepsis and, when present, are indicative of a poor prognosis. The kidneys are particularly sensitive to cytokine-induced damage. Pro-inflammatory cytokines can be produced by renal mesangial, tubular and endothelial cells. Local nitric oxide production is increased, resulting in increased renal blood flow, particularly in the renal medulla. Activation of the coagulation cascade, with the subsequent deposition of fibrin, may also be implicated in sepsis-induced renal dysfunction.

3.2.6 - IMMUNOSUPPRESSION IN THE COURSE OF SEPSIS

Late in the course of sepsis, there is a phase of immunosuppression, which can be a consequence of anergy, lymphopenia, hypothermia and nosocomial infections. The lymphocytes of patients **in** this stage of sepsis, when stimulated **in vitro** with LPS, express a lower quantity of pro-inflammatory cytokines than the lymphocytes of healthy individuals (RUSSEL, 2006). In addition, there is an increase in the apoptosis of circulating lymphocytes and splenic dendritic cells in patients who die from sepsis. While apoptosis is an adaptive response to damaged tissues, it can also contribute to organ dysfunction and immunosuppression in sepsis, thus contributing to the perpetuation of organ dysfunction, long ICU stays and increased mortality **(O'BRIEN** et al., 2007).

3.2.7 - EPIDEMIOLOGY OF SEPSIS

Epidemiological studies of sepsis have been important for notifying the real impact of this pathology on health systems around the world, both from a social and economic point of view. It is a syndrome that has high mortality rates and represents high maintenance costs in ICUs (CARVALHO; TROTTA, 2003; CHALUPKA, TALMOR, 2012). In the United States, according to the **Centre for Disease Control** (CDC), in 1990 there were around 450,000 cases of sepsis per year with more than 100,000 deaths (CDC, 1990). (2001) added important information on the epidemiology of sepsis in that country. In this study, there were 3 cases of severe sepsis per 1,000 inhabitants, and 2.26 cases per 100 hospital discharges. Of the approximately 751,000 cases of severe sepsis in the study, almost 70 per cent (513,000) received intensive care. The estimated mortality rate was 28.5 per cent, or a total of 215,000 deaths nationwide, and the average cost per case was $22,100, with a total annual cost of $16.7 billion. [a] In 2002, the CDC published a report considering sepsis to be the 10th leading cause of death, accounting for 1.3% of deaths that year (ANDERSON, 2002; JAIMES, 2005).

In European countries, the epidemiological studies reported show a wide variation in incidence and mortality rates, reflecting different decision-making in the collection of results, as well as differences in data collection procedures or methodological approaches. A French multicentre study showed a high incidence of septic shock with 8.2 cases per 100 hospitalisations associated with a mortality rate of 60.1% (ANNANE et al., 2003). A study approved by the European Society of Intensive Care, involving nine institutions in 24 countries, revealed a mortality rate ranging from 14% to 41% in hospital units and 8% to 35% in ICUs. This report shows a correlation between multiple organ failure and mortality in critically ill patients with sepsis (VINCENT et al., 2006). In Latin America, Jaimes (2005) reviewed 20 epidemiological studies published between 1994 and 2000 on sepsis and severe sepsis from Argentina, Bolivia, Brazil, Chile, Colombia, Cuba, Ecuador and Mexico, warning that clinical and epidemiological approaches have sometimes been inadequate in terms of research designs, study population and clinical outcome.

In Brazil, the BASES study - Brazilian Sepsis Epidemiology Study, between 2001 and 2002, carried out in five ICUs in the south and southeast regions, found mortality rates of 11% for SIRS, 33.9% for sepsis, 46.9% for severe sepsis and 52.2% for septic shock (SILVA et al., 2004). Sales et al. (2006) analysed data from 75 ICUs in different regions and found mortality rates of 16.7% for sepsis, 34% for severe sepsis and 65.3% for septic shock. Currently, it is believed that around 30 million sepsis-related cases occur every year, with a mortality rate of one in four people, and an increasing incidence rate of one in five. It exceeds the mortality rate of classic diseases such as ischaemic stroke, acute myocardial infarction and is responsible for more deaths than bowel and breast cancer combined. It accounts for 25 per cent of ICU bed occupancy in the country and is the leading cause of death in the ICU
(VIANA, 2011; DELLINGER et al., 2013). According to data from the Latin American Sepsis Institute (DELLINGER, et al., 2013), in a study carried out between 2005 and 2013, 14,643 patients in Brazil were found to have sepsis; of these, 55.2 per cent had severe sepsis and 44.8 per cent had septic shock, with mortality rates of 34.8 per cent and 64.5 per cent respectively (DELLINGER, et al., 2013). As well as being a serious public health problem, sepsis is also a financial problem, since its treatment requires a long stay in the ICU, in addition to the use of expensive antibiotics (KOENIG, 2010). The choice of these antibiotics and other therapeutic measures in sepsis represents a challenge for medicine, since sepsis still remains an entity that

is difficult to manage clinically, due to the haemodynamic and hydroelectrolytic alterations resulting from this state. In this sense, interventions that seek to reduce morbidity and mortality and improve the prognosis of patients with sepsis have been extensively investigated (SIQUEIRA- BATISTA, 2011).

3.2.8 - ACUTE LUNG INJURY

A possible consequence of septicaemia is acute lung injury, a local response to multiple systemic stimuli in the lung, the pathogenesis of which remains unclear (BRODY, 2006). Stimulation of the innate immune system, activation of white blood cells and the response of endothelial cells can lead to the release of a number of mediators or cytokines. This activation causes a variety of physiological changes including vasodilation, an increase in adhesion molecules, an increase in capillary permeability, an increase in clot formation and a decrease in fibrinolysis. Although the immune system response is protective in nature, designed to fight infection in sepsis, hyperactivity of mediators has been cited as a causal factor contributing to endothelial cell damage, microcapillary permeability changes, capillary extravasation, profound vasodilation and hypotension (KLEINPELL et al., 2013).

According to Silva and Abreu (2011) acute lung injury (ALI) results from diseases with direct injury to the alveolar epithelium (pulmonary ALI), such as pneumonia and gastric aspiration, but also from indirect injury (extrapulmonary ALI), i.e. subsidiary to a systemic inflammatory response that primarily damages the capillary endothelium, as in sepsis. The lungs are a common site of injury. ALI is one of the manifestations of lung damage that occurs during sepsis and SIRS (JOHNSON et al., 2004; BOLLER; OTTO, 2009). The pathophysiology of ALI includes damage to the alveoli and pulmonary endothelium, causing extravasation of fluid from blood vessels, generating pulmonary oedema, which then impairs gas exchange in these cases. Lung damage in sepsis occurs as a result of the action of inflammatory mediators such as reactive oxygen molecules and metabolites arachidonic acid and cytokines (JOHNSON et al., 2004).

ALI is characterised by a ratio between the partial pressure of oxygen in arterial blood (PaO_2) and the inspiratory oxygen fraction (FIO_2) < 300 mmHg, bilateral and diffuse pulmonary infiltrates, absence of a cardiogenic component in the genesis of pulmonary oedema (pulmonary capillary wedge pressure < 18 mmHg), presence of risk factors such as shock, sepsis, systemic inflammatory response and intra-abdominal infection/inflammation (COIMBRA et al. 18 mmHg), presence of risk factors such as shock, sepsis, systemic inflammatory response and intra-abdominal infection/inflammation (COIMBRA et al., 2001). Approximately 20% of patients with severe sepsis develop pulmonary dysfunction (LUCAS, 2007), and the deleterious effects of tissue injury, according to Wheeler (1999), are potentiated by various organ characteristics. These include their greater exposure to exogenous agents, the presence of tissue macrophages, the blood pathway, microvasculature and high tissue perfusion. Thus, the primary focus of gram-negative sepsis is the lungs, kidneys and gastrointestinal system. For this reason, sepsis-induced acute lung injury (ALI) remains a major clinical problem with significant morbidity and mortality.

According to an epidemiological, prospective, observational study carried out by Barreto et al. (2016) involving all adult patients admitted or diagnosed with severe sepsis or septic shock in the Urgency and Emergency Department of a public university hospital in southern Brazil, between August 2013 and August 2014, in a total of 95 patients, the infection rate per patient showed a predominance of the pulmonary focus (n=73; 76.8%). According to Yurdakoc (2008), neutrophils contribute significantly to the pathophysiological characteristics of acute lung injury, as does the protein-rich fluid exudate that crosses the endothelial-alveolar-capillary barrier. There is evidence that the production of nitric oxide and pro-inflammatory cytokines play a pivotal role in changes in circulation and tissue injury in pathologies such as sepsis and septic shock (KAOET, et al., 2007). Reverón (2000) observes that during IPA, alveolar macrophages act by releasing cytokines that activate the coagulation and complement systems, enabling the metabolism of arachidonic acid, plasma proteases and oxidants, which in turn cause histological damage to the tissue parenchyma.

The lungs are involved early on in the inflammatory process that occurs in sepsis. Acute lung injury is characterised by neutrophil activation, interstitial oedema, loss of pulmonary surfactant and fibrin-rich alveolar exudate. Post-mortem studies have shown that these alterations are more marked on the epithelial side of the alveolar-capillary membrane, with apoptosis and cell necrosis being possible causes.

Clark (2006) reports that in recent decades, studies have pointed to the numerous mediators of inflammation, such as cytokines, chemokines and leucocytes, as being responsible for this dysfunction. Sepsis has been considered a severe immunological response, and some general anaesthetics, such as propofol, ketamine, isofluorane and urethane have been shown to suppress pro-inflammatory cytokines and iNOS activity, as well as increasing survival rates in murine models (KRUMHOLZ, et al., 1999; GALLEY, et al., 1998; TANIGUCHI, et al., 2001). With regard to surgical interventions, there has also been a gradual increase in the incidence of sepsis and acute lung injury. Currently, these interventions make use of general anaesthesia, the main purpose of which is to promote a reversible condition of comfort, immobility and physiological stability in the patient, which is essential before and after a surgical procedure (GILMAN, 2005), with propofol, sevofluorane and isofluorane being widely used for this purpose.

In their study, De Blasi et al. (2008) point out that general anaesthetics are known to alter microcirculation, probably influencing the onset of acute lung injury. With the increase in the number of cases of this pathology, there are proposals to formulate drugs that guarantee more safety for patients in terms of controlling inflammation, because they would be more effective in their proposed effect. One of the best-known processes, and the one most involved in tissue damage induced by the inflammatory response, is neutrophil migration. Taking lung injury as an example, neutrophil migration is induced by chemokines from the vasculature of the lungs into the alveoli, involving neutrophils passing through the endothelium, the interstitial matrix and the cell junctions that join the alveolar epithelium. Thus, neutrophils can damage the alveolar clearance mechanism and thus fill the alveoli with fluids in conditions characterised as pulmonary inflammation or acute lung injury, compromising gas exchange, especially oxygen (less soluble than CO2).According to Sales (2006), these findings indicate that anaesthesia and surgery themselves trigger a pulmonary inflammatory response, since in both phenomena, the body's haemodynamics, as well as perfusion and microvasculature are altered. To this end, pro-inflammatory cytokines are the most important contributing factors in potentiating inflammation, and it is likely that the production of these cytokines by alveolar macrophages contributes to the influx of neutrophils and macrophage aggregation. In this event, neutrophils or polymorphonuclear leucocytes (PMNs) play an important role in the inflammatory response, both in sepsis and in bronchopulmonary dysplasia and acute lung injury (ABRAHAN, 2003), as they are essential in the host's first defence mechanism against infection. The balance of chemokines produced locally by macrophages and others produced away from the site of inflammation are important for directing neutrophil migration to the lungs (CHOPRA, 2009).

In response to this chemical gradient, neutrophils cross the endothelium and release numerous proteolytic enzymes and reactive oxygen species after recruitment to the infection site.

Paradoxically, this event also stimulates the release of interleukin 10 (IL-10), which is an anti-inflammatory modulator of the immune response. It has been suggested that the production of IL-10 by macrophages occurs after the phagocytosis of dead neutrophils. In turn, IL-10 may subsequently suppress additional cytokine production and the phagocytic activity of alveolar macrophages, allowing neutrophils to serve both a pro- and anti-inflammatory capacity in this situation (REDDY et al., 2001). In order to induce and potentiate the inflammatory response, alveolar macrophages also release cell mediators such as tumour necrosis factor (TNF), interferon gamma (IFN) and eicosanoids (PGE2) during the initial phase of lung inflammation (CHOPRA, 2009).

When there is damage to the alveolar-capillary membrane, regardless of the cause triggering the lung injury, with extravasation of protein-rich fluid into the alveolar space. Alveolar epithelial damage involves the basal membrane and type I and II pneumocytes, leading to a reduction in the quantity and altered functionality of surfactant, with a consequent increase in alveolar surface tension, the occurrence of atelectasis and a reduction in lung compliance. Injury to the capillary endothelium is associated with numerous inflammatory events, such as recruitment, sequestration and activation of neutrophils; formation of oxygen radicals; activation of the coagulation system, leading to microvascular thrombosis; and recruitment of mesenchymal cells, with the production of procollagen. In the alveolar space, the balance between pro-inflammatory mediators (TNF-α, IL-1, IL-6 and IL-8) and anti-inflammatory mediators (IL-10, IL-1 receptor antagonists and soluble TNF receptor antagonists) favours the maintenance of inflammation. Initial lung damage is followed by repair, remodelling and fibrosing alveolitis (WARE, 2006).

The impact on respiratory function due to changes in respiratory mechanics caused by acute or chronic inflammation is well described in the literature (PETÁK et al., 2002; MACEDO-NETO et al., 1998). It is known that, among other dysfunctions, increased pulmonary vascular permeability leads to pulmonary oedema, which causes changes in pulmonary compliance and pulmonary elastance (PARKER et al., 1999; PETÁK et al., 2002).

CHAPTER 4

MATERIALS AND METHODS

This study was approved by the Ethics Committee for the Use of Animals of the Federal University of Rio Grande do Norte (CEUA - UFRN), under protocol number No. 052/2014.

All experimental procedures are in accordance with the **Guide for the Care and Use of** Laboratory Animals (*USA - National Research Council*) and COBEA (Colégio Brasileiro de Experimentação Animal).

4.1 - OBTAINING THE MICROEMULSION SYSTEM (ME)

The first stage of the experimental work consisted of obtaining the microemulsion system that was used. The choice of microemulsion was made by constructing the ternary diagram, which made it possible to visualise the behaviour of the system's phases by varying the concentrations of its components. The method used was based on volumetric titration with analytical weighing of the v/v proportions, in order to obtain the respective mass proportions (RAMOS, 1996). To construct the diagram, various proportions were weighed out in the binary active material (surfactant), for this study soya lecithin was used, and the aqueous component (5% ethanol solution), then titration was started with the oily component (bullfrog oil), describing the phase transitions by visual observation, after stirring and centrifuging the sample. Phase equilibrium was characterised using the Winsor classification (1948).

4.2 - EXPERIMENTAL MODEL

4.2.1 - MUMMIES

To carry out the experiments, **Mus musculus Swiss** mice, with an average age of 35±5 days, males, weighing around 30g±5, were used as an experimental model.

4.2.2 - STUDY DESIGN

The mice were initially selected at random, placed in polypropylene cages and divided into three groups: (1) negative control (saline solution), (2) positive control (frog oil) and (3) experimental group (microemulsion). The animals were kept under ideal conditions of temperature (22 ± 3^0 C) and humidity (50 ± 20%), with controlled lighting on a 12-hour light/dark regime, and given water and feed (Labina, Purina®) **ad libitum**. All the animals used in this study came from the vivarium of the University Centre of Rio Grande do Norte - UNI-RN.

For all groups, a total volume of 100 pl/day was administered by gavage, with 0.9% saline solution for the negative control, frog oil for the positive control and the microemulsion for the experimental group.

For the experimental sepsis model, the animals received a pre-treatment for a period of 30 consecutive and uninterrupted days. On the 30th day after administration of the solutions, all the animals in each group were operated on using the CLP (**caecal ligation puncture)** technique to induce sub-lethal sepsis.

For the experimental muscle injury model, the animals were pre-treated for 4 consecutive and uninterrupted days. After this period, the animals underwent induction of muscle damage by inoculating the right gastrocnemius muscle belly with 10% formalin.

4.2.3 - EVALUATION OF THE TOXICITY POTENTIAL OF PURE AND MICROEMULSIFIED BULLFROG OIL

The toxicity of pure and microemulsified bullfrog oil was analysed by ingesting the substances every day for 15 consecutive days. At the end, liver tissue samples were taken from the animals and histologically analysed to check for signs of tissue damage.

4.2.4 - SEPSIS INDUCTION

Sepsis was induced according to the methodology described by Baker et al. (1983), with some modifications. To this end, an incision of approximately 1.0 cm was made in the cranial-caudal axis of the animals' abdomens, reaching the abdominal cavity and exposing the caecum (first portion of the large intestine). The caecal appendix (vermiform) was perforated by passing it through with a 21G needle so that faeces could leak into the abdominal cavity and consequently induce sepsis. The skin and peritoneum were then sutured and the animals were exposed to light in order to control their temperature and avoid hypothermia. For the procedure, the animals were anaesthetised with the inhalation anaesthetic sevofluorane using the Oxigel 717/0101 inhalation anaesthesia machine, ventilator 1530.

4.2.5 - ANALYSIS OF THE SURVIVAL RATE OF SEPTIC MICE TREATED WITH PURE AND MICROEMULSIFIED BULLFROG OIL

The survival rate of the animals was based on daily ingestion of the substances (pure bullfrog oil, microemulsion and saline) by gavage for 30 consecutive days. At the end of this time, the animals in each group (n=10) were subjected to sepsis induction using the CLP technique. After this induction, the animals were observed daily, with behavioural patterns and resistance to sepsis recorded.

4.2.6 - BRONCHOALVEOLAR LAVAGE (LBA)

To analyse the migration of cells into the animals' lungs, an opening was made in the trachea and a cannula with 1.0 ml of sterile saline solution was inserted, injecting a volume until the lungs were inflated to the maximum. The aspirates were then placed in sterile **Eppendorf** tubes for subsequent centrifugation and cell counting in a Neubauer chamber.

4.2.7 - ANALYSIS OF THE ANTI-EDEMATOGENIC ACTIVITY OF PURE AND MICROEMULSIFIED BULLFROG OIL

To induce muscle inflammation, 100 pl of the solutions were administered over 4 consecutive days using the gavage technique. Once the pre-treatment had been completed, the animals were anaesthetised by inhalation for subsequent induction of muscle damage, with the inoculation of 20 µl of 10% formalin into the animals' gastrocnemius muscle. The lesion was assessed based on the horizontal extension of the muscle (oedema), using a digital caliper, always positioned in the middle third of the animal's leg. The extent of the lesions was checked at intervals of 5 minutes, 1, 2, 3, 4, 5 and 24 hours after induction. For histological analysis, dissections were made of the gastrocnemius muscle to assess the presence of tissue damage.

4.2.8   - HISTOPATHOLOGICAL ANALYSIS OF THE SAMPLES

The biopsy samples from the lung, liver and muscle tissues were removed and fixed in 10% formalin solution. All the samples were embedded in paraffin, cut on a microtome and the slides prepared and stained using the haematoxylin-eosin (HE) technique. At the end of the process, the slides were photographed with a digital camera and the images captured and processed by the manufacturer's software for detailed visualisation of the tissues.

4.2.9 - STATISTICAL ANALYSES

SigmaStat v 3.10 was used for the statistical analyses of the results, where analysis of variance **(ANOVA)** was carried out for non-parametric data (Kruskal-Wallis). When statistically significant differences were found, the **Student-Newman-Keuls post-hoc** test was used for multiple comparison of means.

CHAPTER 5

RESULTS AND DISCUSSION

5.1   - OBTAINING AND CHARACTERISING THE SYSTEM

MICROEMULSIFIED

The chemical substances used to construct the phase diagram were analysed for their solubility in the polar phase (alcohol solution) and the oil phase (Rana catesbeiana oil) at room temperature of 28° C. This study resulted in a diagram containing soya lecithin as the surfactant, Rana catesbeiana oil as the oil phase and a 70 % ethanol solution (figure 11).

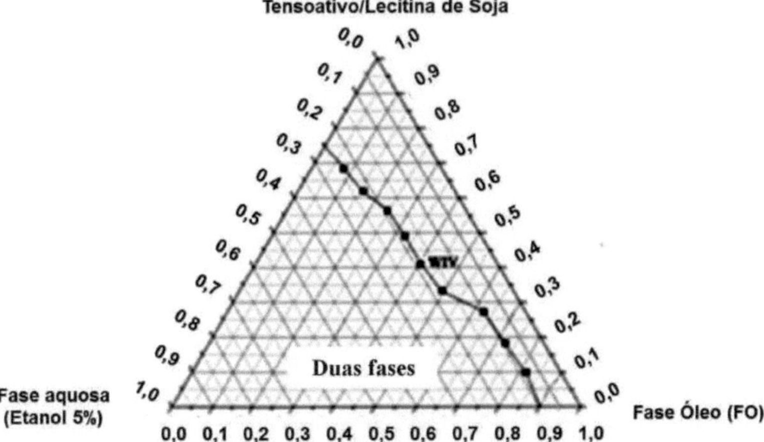

Figura 12:   Ternary diagram of the system: T = soya lecithin; FO = pure Rana catesbeiana oil and FA = 70 % aqueous ethanol solution.

The diagram shows the region of interest, which is the microemulsion (WIV). For this diagram, the polar phase is a 70% alcohol solution (ethanol), which has a lower polarity than distilled water, causing the hydrophilic part of the soya lecithin (surfactant) to interact with the aqueous phase, thus favouring the accommodation of the surfactant molecule at the water-oil interface (A/O) and the formation of micellar aggregates, i.e. the formation of the microemulsion.

5.2 - ANALYSIS OF THE TOXICITY OF PURE AND MICROEMULSIFIED BULLFROG OIL.

To analyse the toxicity potential of pure and microemulsified bullfrog oil, the animals were given 100p l of the respective substances every day for 15 consecutive and uninterrupted days. Because bullfrog oil contains polyunsaturated fatty acids and is metabolised in the liver, samples of this tissue were taken for histopathological analysis to assess signs of hepatotoxicity in the animals in the groups treated with pure bullfrog oil and microemulsion.

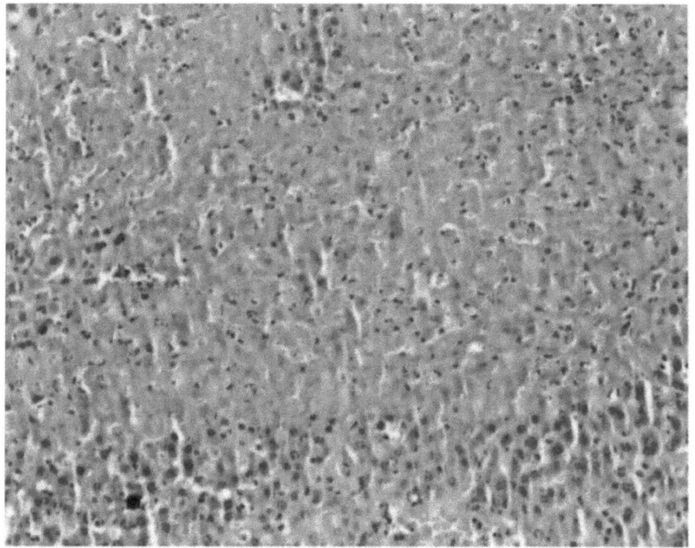

Image 1: Histological section of liver tissue from an animal in the microemulsion group (100x magnification).

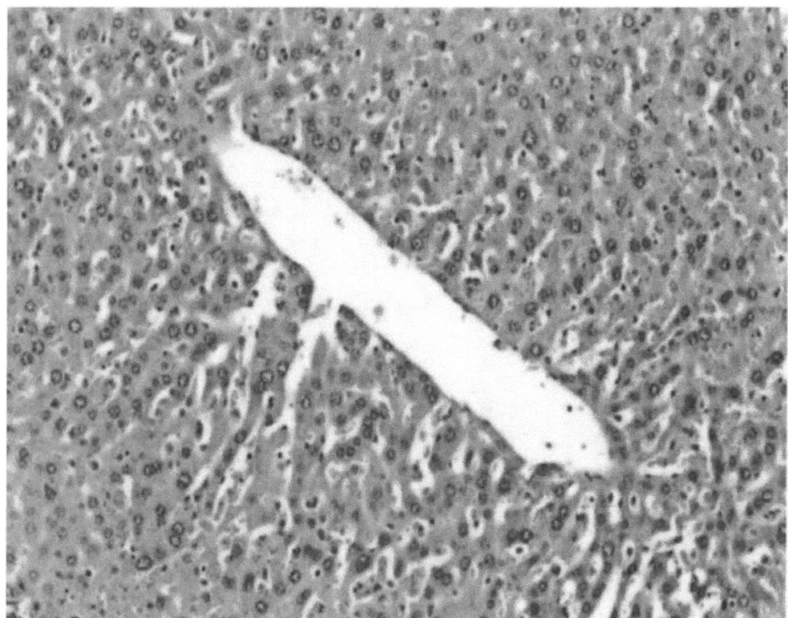

Image 2: Histological section of liver tissue from an animal in the microemulsion group (100x magnification).

The results show that in the group in which the microemulsion (ME) was administered, the liver's architecture was preserved, with no signs of fibrosis, but with foci of hepatocytic necrosis accompanied by polymorphonuclear infiltrates, subcapsular coagulative necrosis and sinusoidal dilatation in zone 3, which shows a clinical picture of hepatic steatosis (Images 1 and 2).

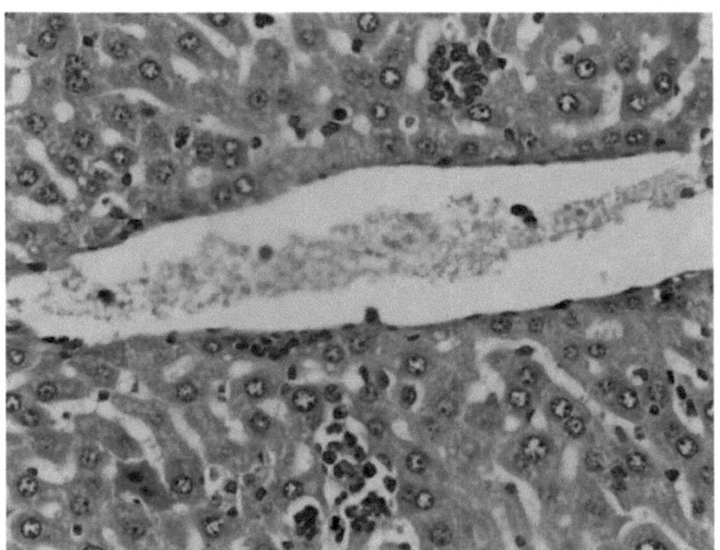

Image 3: Histological section of liver tissue from animals in the pure bullfrog oil group (400x magnification).

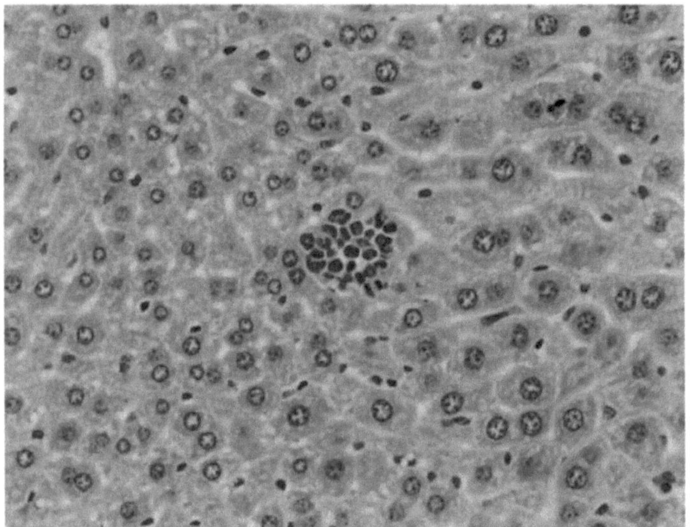

Image 4: Histological section of liver tissue from animals in the pure bullfrog oil group (400x magnification).

In the group given pure bullfrog oil, multiple foci of hepatocytic necrosis were observed, accompanied by polymorphonuclear infiltrates, showing hepatocytes with microvesicular steatosis (zones 2 and 3), acidophilia, tumefaction and binucleation. These findings show steatohepatitis, i.e. a more advanced stage in relation to hepatic steatosis and a precursor to hepatic carcinoma (Images 3 and 4).

The results obtained show that bullfrog oil in microemulsion was able to attenuate the hepatotoxic potential when compared to pure oil. Substances with possible therapeutic potential for pharmaceutical formulations need to be subjected to toxicity analyses, such as genotoxicity and cytotoxicity tests.

In the study by Amaral-Machado 2016, it was observed that bullfrog oil in a nanostructured system presented itself as a potential candidate for drug development, as it is free of toxicity and very effective in antineoplastic therapy. These data corroborate the findings of this study, highlighting pure bullfrog oil and its use in micro and nanostructured systems as an animal product with significant and promising therapeutic potential.

12.3   - ANALYSIS OF THE SURVIVAL RATE OF SEPTIC MICE TREATED WITH PURE AND MICROEMULSIFIED BULLFROG OIL.

For 30 days, 100µl of saline solution (control group), pure bullfrog oil (OR) and microemulsion (ME) were administered orally by gavage. At the end of the period, the animals in each group (n=10) were submitted to a septic condition using the CLP technique, in order to analyse their survival rates.

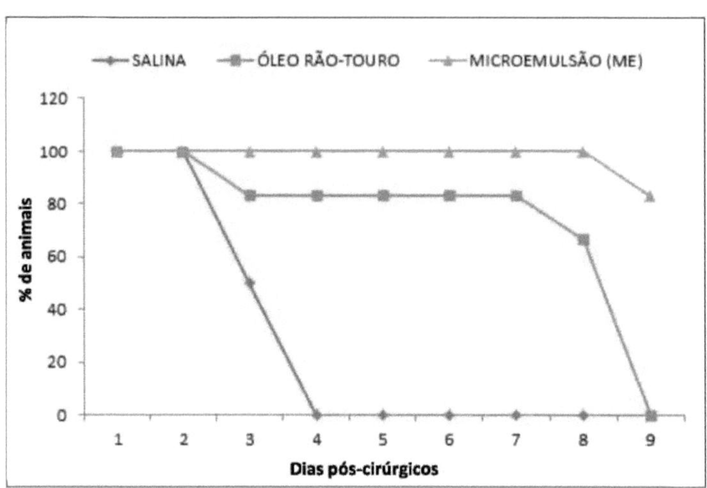

Figura 13: Analysis of the survival rate of septic mice treated with pure bullfrog oil and in microemulsion.

As can be seen in figure 12, the negative control group (saline) showed mortality in all the animals by the fourth day after sepsis, with mortality beginning in the first 48 hours. This behaviour is expected due to the intense systemic inflammatory response and, as it is a "placebo" group, it does not act on the response and consequently does not protect the animals from severe sepsis and subsequent progression to septic shock. On the other hand, the group treated with pure bullfrog oil showed total mortality of the animals by the ninth day post-sepsis, with the first deaths being observed from the first 72 hours after induction of the septic condition. In the group treated with ME, animals (n=2) died only on the eighth day after sepsis induction, with a survival rate of 80 per cent. In this group, no mortality was observed until the eighth day of sepsis induction. Figure 12 shows the behaviour of this study.

5.4 - EVALUATION OF LEUKOCYTE MIGRATION TO THE LUNGS THROUGH BRONCHOALVEOLAR LAVAGE IN SEPTIC MICE

In this study, 100μl/day of pure bullfrog oil and microemulsion were administered orally via gavage for 30 days without interruption. After this period, a septic condition was induced in the animals using the same technique as CLP and, after 8 hours, bronchoalveolar lavage (BAL) was carried out and the number of cells determined by counting them in a

Neubauer chamber. Figure 13 shows the results obtained in this study.

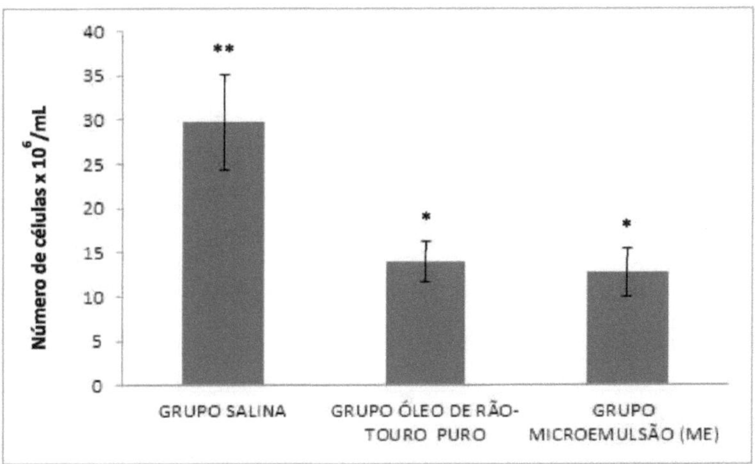

Figura 14: Evaluation of cell migration to the lungs after sepsis induction. ** P ≤ 0.001; * P > 0.05

The results obtained in figure 13 show that in the septic animals given saline solution (negative control), there was an intense migration of neutrophils to the lung tissue. When cell migration was analysed in the groups treated with pure bullfrog oil and in microemulsion, a statistically significant reduction (P ≤ 0.001) in cell migration was observed when compared to the negative control group. When the pure bullfrog oil and microemulsion groups were compared, no statistically significant difference was observed (**P** > 0.05).

There is currently no effective pharmacological treatment for acute lung injury and the resulting acute respiratory distress syndrome. Some studies are looking for substances of animal and plant origin that act on acute lung injury, in order to reduce the intensity of the inflammatory response and the installation of lesions (injuries), characteristic of the post-septic condition, because during sepsis there are significant vascular changes that alter the permeability of the microvasculature and potentiate the wear and tear of heavily perfused organs such as the lungs, brain and kidneys. The excess migration of leucocytes to these organs ends up increasing the release of proteolytic enzymes into the tissue, leading to wear and tear and impairment of the organ. In the study by Yali Zhang et al. (2015), 30 analogues of curcumin, extracted from turmeric, were analysed using a biosynchronisation assay and most of the compounds inhibited the LPS-induced production of TNF and IL-6. The active compounds, a17, a18, c9 and c26, displayed their anti-inflammatory activity **in** a dose-dependent manner and exhibited greater stability than curcumin **in vitro**. In addition, the active compound c26 dose-dependently inhibited ERK phosphorylation.

In vivo, LPS significantly increased the concentration of proteins and the number of inflammatory cells in bronchoalveolar lavage, lung oedema, pathological changes in lung tissue, inflammatory cytokines in serum and lavage, macrophage infiltration, expression of inflammatory genes and phosphorylation of MAPKs. However, pretreatment with c26 attenuated the LPS-induced increase via the ERK pathway **in vivo**. However, this same study showed that the instability of curcumin limits its clinical application. The results observed in these tests corroborate the findings of this study with pure bullfrog oil and in a microemulsion system, since the use of pure oil limits its clinical application, as it has good anti-inflammatory potential but leads to tissue injury. When it is present in the formulation of a microemulsified system, the concentration of the oil is reduced and no significant lung damage is observed.

In the study by Takashima et al. (2014), the anti-inflammatory and antioxidant activities of quercetin, which is one of the most common flavonoids found in fruits and vegetables, were evaluated. In this study, it was investigated whether intratracheal administration of quercetin could suppress acute lung injury (ALI) induced by lipopolysaccharide (LPS) in rats, as well as the involvement of HO-1 in the suppressive effects of quercetin. Intratracheal administration of quercetin decreased the weight ratio

in relation to the body. In addition, quercetin decreased myeloproteinase (MMP-9) activity and the production of pro-inflammatory cytokines in bronchoalveolar lavage cells activated by LPS. Thus, it was observed that quercetin exhibits important cytoprotective effects through the induction of heme oxygenase (HO)-1, thus preventing the installation of relevant lung lesions, similar to the findings when evaluating bullfrog oil in a microemulsion system.

14.5 - HISTOPATHOLOGICAL ANALYSIS OF THE LUNG TISSUE OF SEPTIC MICE.

Eight hours after the induction of the septic condition, the animals treated with pure bullfrog oil and in microemulsion were euthanised for the subsequent removal of lung tissue samples and histopathological analyses (Images 5 and 6). In all the samples analysed from the OR-treated animals, an exacerbated migration of leukocytes to the lungs was observed, with the presence of cellular infiltrate (resulting pulmonary oedema), rupture of alveolar walls with diffuse alveolar damage, typical of the cascade process of chronic lesion development. The histological analyses observed in this group indicate the onset of a significant case of acute lung injury (IPA).

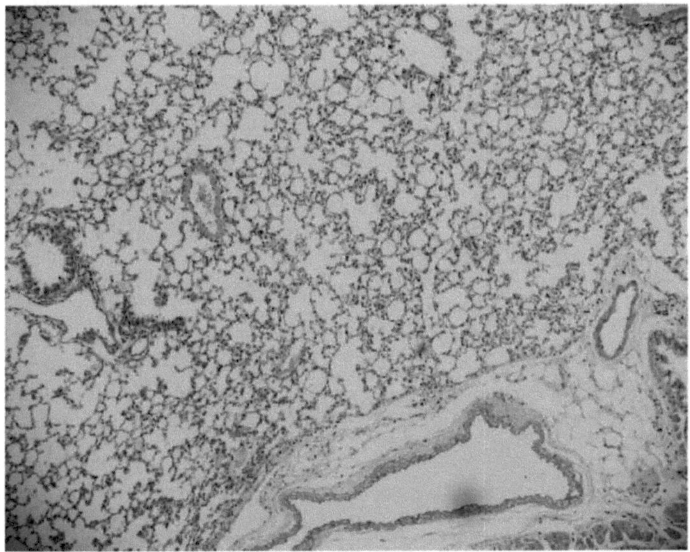

Image 5: Histological section of lung tissue from animals in the pure bullfrog oil group.
Early exudative stage with hyaline membranes outlining alveolar spaces and interstitial oedema **(original magnification 200x).**

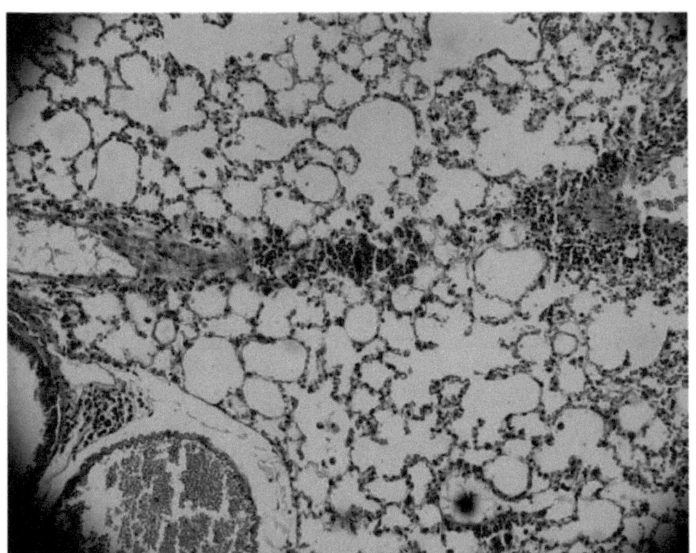

Image 6: Histological section of lung tissue from animals in the pure bullfrog oil group. Late exudative / proliferative phase **(original magnification 200x).**

In all the samples analysed, the animals treated with the microemulsion showed greater lung tissue integrity, with reduced leukocyte migration and a consequent reduction in cellular infiltrate (pulmonary oedema) and tissue damage, as shown in images 7 and 8. When compared to the group treated with pure bullfrog oil, there was less wear and tear of the lung parenchyma in the samples from the animals treated with the microemulsion.

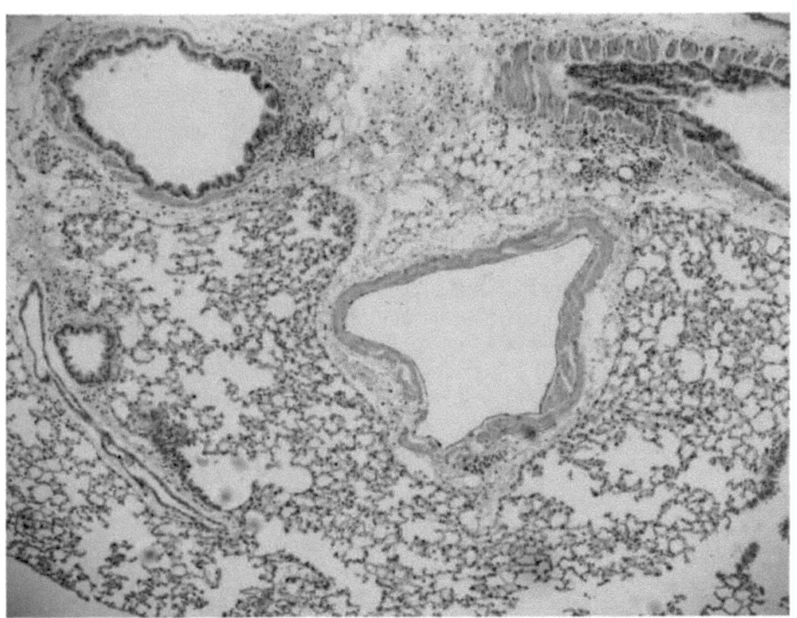

Image 7: Histological section of lung tissue from an animal in the microemulsion group.

Presence of intact hyaline membranes and absence of alveolar spaces and interstitial oedema **(original magnification 200x).**

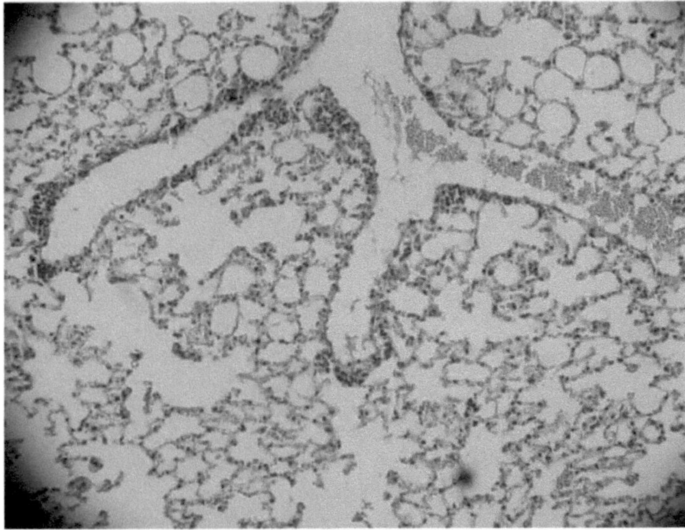

Image 8: Histological section of lung tissue from an animal in the microemulsion group.

Presence of partially intact hyaline membranes and few alveolar spaces and absence of interstitial oedema **(original magnification 200x).**

Acute lung injury (ALI) and acute respiratory distress syndrome (ARDS) are a continuum of alterations resulting from a wide variety of lung injuries, often resulting in significant morbidity and frequent death. Studies into the molecular pathophysiology of the course of IPA/ARDS are still unclear, but more recent studies aim to develop molecular biomarkers that will improve the prognosis of the disease and therapeutic management (BUTT et al., 2016). As most cases of IPA/ARDS are diagnosed clinically and radiographically, biopsies (histopathological analyses) are rarely requested for diagnosis, largely because it is an invasive process and poses risks to the patient. Biopsies are typically performed in cases where the presentation is not straightforward, a specific infection is being considered or the therapeutic response is disappointing (GAJIC et al., 2011). Diffuse alveolar damage, i.e. rupture of the alveolar wall, usually occurs as the culmination of the IPA cascade process, developing from epithelial barrier dysfunction, endothelial dysfunction (due to increased permeability of the microvasculature) and resulting pulmonary infiltrate (oedema). As described by Katzenstein (2006), diffuse alveolar damage can be divided into 3 phases: acute, early or exudative; organising or proliferative, and late resolution or fibrotic phase, which represents the most severe stage of the condition. The acute phase is characterised by distinctive hyaline membranes that line alveolar spaces. Images 5 and 6 show this finding in the animals treated with pure bullfrog oil, with an intense cellular infiltrate (oedema), corroborating the findings in the literature. Endothelial cells and pneumocytes suffer necrosis. The hyaline membranes begin to organise as the DAD continues in the organisation phase and granulation tissue develops in the alveolar spaces. In individuals who survive a septic condition, it is common to observe respiratory alterations. In many cases, these are due to changes in the microvascular permeability of the lungs, the target organ for this type of injury due to its intense vascularisation. In his studies, Douda (2011) states that in the lungs, activated neutrophils produce numerous cytotoxic substances, including pro-inflammatory cytokines, reactive oxygen species, bioactive lipids, as well as various granular enzymes. Specifically, these enzymes wear down the hyaline membranes that make up the lung parenchyma, causing serious damage to the walls of the alveoli. The resulting pulmonary oedema impairs gas exchange, which in some cases can lead to respiratory failure and even death.

5.6 - EVALUATION OF THE ANTI-OEDEMATOGENIC POTENTIAL OF PURE AND MICROEMULSIFIED BULLFROG OIL.

As illustrated in Figure 14, when the microemulsion and negative control groups (saline) are compared, a statistically significant difference can be observed (p <0.001). When the microemulsion and pure bullfrog oil groups are compared, there is no statistically significant difference (p = 0.9027), showing that the microemulsion with an oil concentration of 60% and pure bullfrog oil provide the same efficiency in reducing oedema. When the efficiency of the microemulsion is compared to pure frog oil at the intervals of the measurements, both proved to be effective up to the second hour, where a greater statistical difference is observed with the negative control group, indicating a lesser extent of oedema in both groups. No statistical difference was observed from the third to the twenty-fourth hour after injury induction.

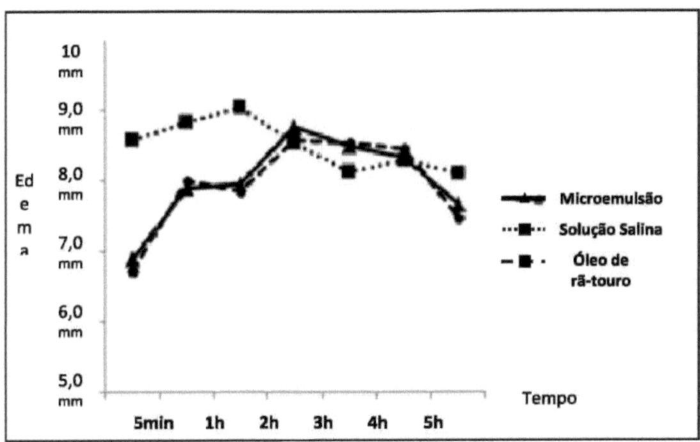

Figura 15: Evaluation of leg oedema induced by 10% formalin in mice treated with pure bullfrog oil and microemulsion.

In the analysis of the oedema caused by the induction of muscle damage in the animals, it was observed that both the microemulsion and pure bullfrog oil showed similar biological activity, significantly reducing oedema in the first few hours when compared to the control group which received only saline solution. This indicates that both microemulsion and pure bullfrog oil have the potential to be used in the treatment of acute inflammation, since they acted effectively in the first hours of the inflammatory response.

When the muscle tissue samples were analysed (images 9 and 10), significant morphological differences were observed in the tissue samples from the microemulsion and pure bullfrog oil groups. There was a slight presence of oedema (cell infiltration) and small signs of tissue damage in the microemulsion group. In the analysis of muscle tissue from the pure bullfrog oil group, there was a significant presence of oedema (cellular infarction) and fragmentation of muscle fibres, indicating the installation of significant muscle damage, given the involvement of fibres.

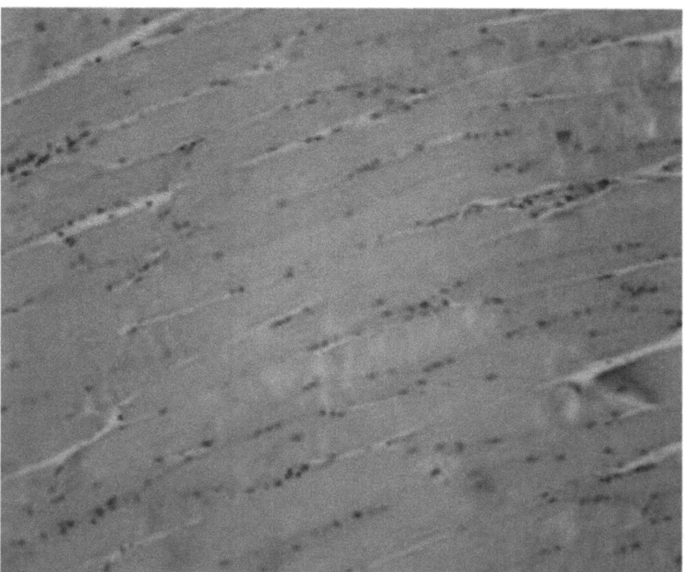

Image 9: Histological section of muscle tissue from animals in the microemulsion group. There

is a slight cellular infiltrate (oedema) and few signs of tissue injury **(original magnification 200x).**

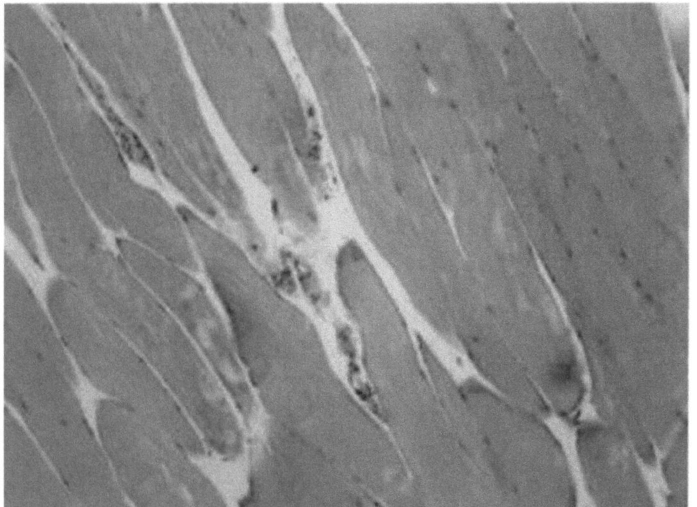

Image 10: Histological section of muscle tissue in animals from the pure bullfrog oil group. Intense muscle oedema and signs of tissue injury can be seen **(original magnification 200x).**

In the histological analysis of the muscle tissue, it is clear that the muscle tissue samples from the animals treated with the pure oil showed a higher level of cellular infiltrate, oedema throughout the tissue and fibre fragmentation. The animals treated with the microemulsion showed a slight cellular infiltrate and oedema, with no damage to the muscle fibres. This leads us to believe that the microemulsion acted to protect the muscle tissue, preventing an exacerbated inflammatory response, certainly due to its greater surface spreading power and interaction with the muscle tissue. Muscle damage is characterised structurally by myofilament rupture, mitochondrial and sarcoplasmic reticulum abnormalities, sarcolemma discontinuity, hydro-electrolytic imbalance and cell necrosis.Histological evidence of tissue injury is related to the number of injured fibres, which are identified using a number of indicators, such as: cellular infiltrate (presence of inflammatory and/or satellite cells); basophilia (increased ribosomal activity); centralised nuclei with prominent nucleoli and hyperconcentration of myofilaments (GORDON et al., 2017), 2017).

Considering that bullfrog oil is rich in polyunsaturated fatty acids and that these are metabolised by the liver, samples of these organs from animals in the microemulsion and pure bullfrog oil groups were taken for macroscopic and histological analyses to check for signs of hepatotoxicity. No damage to the structure of the liver lobes was observed in the microemulsion group, as the hepatocytes had the usual characteristics and sinusoid capillaries were normally positioned radially to the centre of the lobe. The blood vessels had a patent (free) and preserved lumen, with no evidence of any structural damage (Image 11).

Signs of tissue damage were observed in the liver tissue samples from the pure bullfrog oil group. Hepatocyte growth, signs of subscapular necrosis and lesions associated with increased fat absorption by the liver were observed, characterising the hepatotoxic potential of pure bullfrog oil. (Image 12)

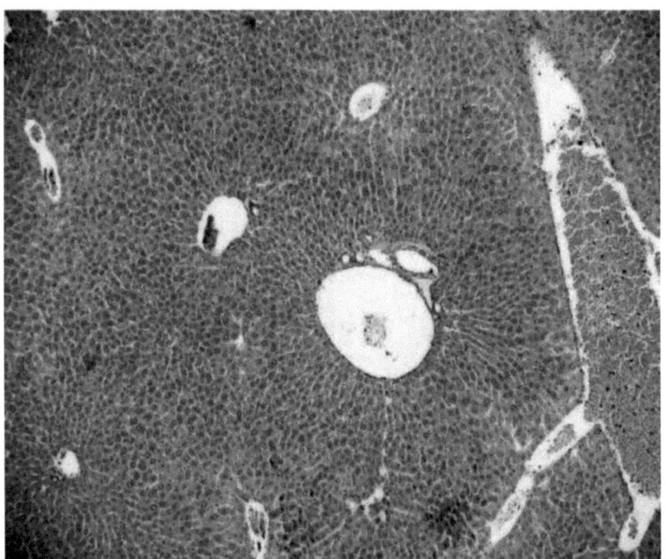

Image 11: Histological section of liver tissue from an animal in the microemulsion group **(original magnification 200x).**

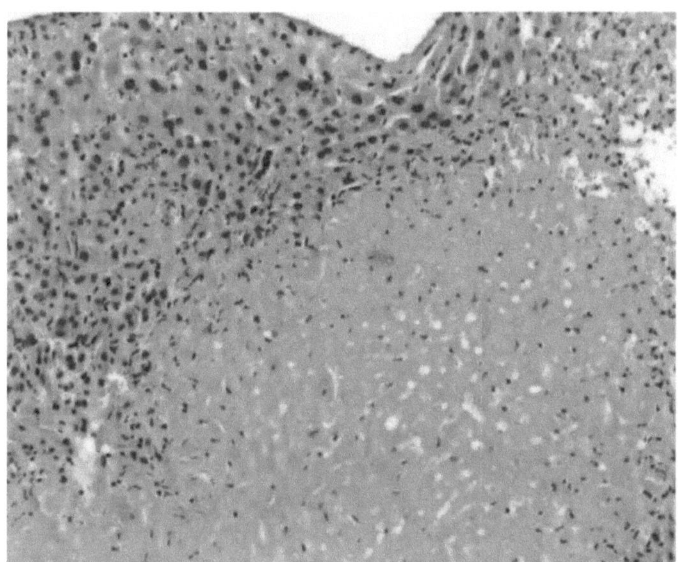

Image 12: Histological section of liver tissue from animals in the pure bullfrog oil group **(original magnification 200x).**

CHAPTER 6

CONCLUSIONS

The results obtained in this study allow us to conclude that:

- It was possible to obtain microemulsion regions with bullfrog oil in compositions compatible with the studies we wanted to carry out.

- The composition of the bullfrog oil microemulsion system tested in this study was: 5% FA, 35% surfactant and 60% oil.

- Both pure and microemulsified bullfrog oil showed anti-inflammatory activity, modulating the inflammatory response.

- The anti-inflammatory activity of microemulsified bullfrog oil proved to be more effective in protecting against the installation of tissue injuries when compared to pure oil.

- The microemulsified oil had no hepatotoxic potential compared to the pure oil, which was highly toxic.

- The microemulsified oil proved to be effective in combating acute septicaemia, increasing the survival rate of the treated group, unlike the group treated with pure oil, where the mortality rate was 80%.

- The microemulsified oil proved to be effective in protecting the lungs, considerably reducing acute lung injury, unlike the treatment with pure oil, which proved incapable of protecting against tissue injury.

- The microemulsified oil proved effective in reducing muscle oedema in the acute phase of inflammation.

With the results obtained, it can be concluded that microemulsified bullfrog oil, containing 60 per cent of the oil phase in its composition, is a new drug delivery system with great viability of application, as it is low cost and easy to access, in the treatment of sepsis and tissue inflammation, without compromising vital organs such as the liver and lungs.

BIBLIOGRAPHICAL REFERENCES

ABBAS A.K.; Murphy K.M.; Sher A. Functional diversity of helper T lymphocytes. **Nature**, v. 383, p. 787-793, Oct., 1996.

ABBAS, A.; LICHTMAN, K. **Cellular and molecular immunology.** 5. ed. Rio de Janeiro: Elsevier, 2005.

ABRAHAM E.; SINGER M. Mechanisms of sepsis-induced organ dysfunction. **Critical Care Medicine**, v. 35, n, 10, p. 2408-16, Oct., 2007.

AGOSTINHO, C.A.; LIMA, S.L.; CASALI, A.P. Zootechnical performance and feed consumption percentage of bullfrogs (**Rana catesbeiana**) in the rearing phase of the amphigranja system. **Revista Brasileira de Zootecnica**, v.32, n.3, p.505-511, 2003.

ANDERSON, R.N.; Deaths: Leading Causes for 2000. **National Vital Statistics Reports**, v. 50, n. 16, Sept., 2002.

ANNANE D.; AEGERTER P.; JARS-GUINCESTRE M.C.; GUIDETFOR B. Current epidemiology of septic shock: The CUB-Réa Network. **American Journal of Respiratory and Critical Care Medicine**, v. 168, n. 2, p. 165-172, Jul., 2003.

AIRD, W.C The role of endothelium in severe sepsis and multiple organ dysfunction syndrome. **Blood**, v. 101, n. 10, p. 3765-77, May, 2003.

ALBERTI, C.; BRUN-Buisson, C.; GOODMAN, S.V. Influence of systemic inflammatory response syndrome and sepsis on outcome of critically ill infected patients. **American Journal of**

Respiratory and Critical Care Medicine, v. 168, n.1, p. 77-84, Jul, 2003.

ANGUS, D.C.; LINDE-ZWIRBLE, W.T.; LIDICKER, J.; CLERMONT, G.; CARCILLO, J.; PINSKY, M.R. Epidemiology of severe sepsis in the United States: analysis of incidence, outcome, and associated costs of care. **Critical Care Medicine**, v.29, n.7, p. 1303-1310, Jul, 2001.

ANGUS, D.C.; PEREIRA, C.A.P.; SILVA, E. Epidemiology of severe sepsis around the world. **Endocrine, Metabolic & Immune Disorders Drug Targets**, v.6, n. 2, p. 207-212, 2006.

BAKER, C.C.; CHAUDRI, I.H.; GAINES, H.O.; BAUER, A.E. Evaluation of factors affecting mortality rate after sepsis in a murine cecal ligation and puncture model. **Surgery**, n.94, v.2, p. 331-335, Aug., 1983.

BALDWIN A. Control of oncogenesis and cancer therapy resistance by the transcription factor NF-kB. - **The Journal Clinicai Investigation**, n. 107, v. 3, p. 241-246, Feb., 2001.

BOELTER, R.A.; CECHIN, S.Z. Impact of the bullfrog diet (Lithobates catesbeianus - Anura, Ranidae) on native fauna: cause study from the region of Agudo RS Brazil. **Natureza & Conservação**, v.5, n.2, p.115-123, Oct., 2007.

BOLLER, E.M.; OTTO, C.M. Septic shoch. In: Silverstein, D. C.; Hopper, K. In: **Small Animal Critical Care Medicine**. St. Louis: Saunders, p. 459-463, 2009.

BONE, R.C.; BALK, R.A.; CERRA, F.B.; DELLINGER, R.P.; FEIN, A.M.; KNAUS, W.A.; SCHEIN, R.M.; SIBBALD, W.J. Definitions for sepsis and oran failure and guidelines for use of innovative therapies in sepsis. The ACCP/SCCM Consensus Conference Committee. American College of Chest Physicians/Society of Critical Care Medicine. **Chest**, v. 101, n.6, p. 1644-1655, 1992a.

BONE, R.C.; IBBALD, W.J.; SPRUNG, C.L. The ACCP-SCCM consensus conference on sepsis and organ failure. **Chest**, v. 101, n.6, p. 1481-1483, 1992b.

BONE, R.C; BALK, R.A; DELLINGER R.P.; FEIN A.M.; KNAUS W.A.; SCHEIN R.M.; SIBBALD, W.J.

American college of chest physicians/society of critical care medicine consensus conference: definitions for sepsis and organ failure and guidelines for the use of innovative therapies in sepsis. **Critical Care Medicine**, v. 20, n. 6, p. 864-874, Jun., 1992

BRODY, T.M.; MINNEMAN, K.P. **Human Pharmacology.** 4. ed. Campus: Elsevier, 2006.

BRUN-BUISSON, C. The epidemiology of the systemic inflammatory response. **Intensive Care Medicine**, v.26, p. 64-74, Jan., 2000.

BRUXEL, F.; LAUX, M.; WILD, L.; FRAGAN, M.; KOESTES, L.S.; TEIXEIRA, H.F. Nanoemulsions as parenteral drug delivery systems. **Química Nova**, v.35, n.9, p. 1827-1840, 2012.

BLASI, R.A.; PALMISANI, S.; BOEZI, M.; ARCIONI, R.; COLLINI, S.; TROISI, F.; PINTO, G. Effects of remifentanil-based general anaesthesia with propofol or sevoflurane on muscle microcirculation as assessed by near-infrared spectroscopy. **Brazilian Journal of Anaesthesiology**, v.101, n. 2 p.171-177, Aug., 2008.

CARVALHO, P.R.A; TROTTA, E.A. Advances in the diagnosis and treatment of sepsis. **Jornal de Pediatria**, v.79, supl. 2, p. 195-204, Nov., 2003.

CASANOVA, M. A.; MEDEIROS, F. Recent evidence on polyunsaturated fatty acids of the omega-3 family in cardiovascular disease. **Revista do Hospital Universitário Pedro Ernesto**, v.1, n. 11, p.74-80, 2011.

CATENACCI M.H.; King K. Severe sepsis and septic shock: improving outcomes in the emergency department. **Emergency Medical Clinics of North America,** v. 26, p. 603-623, 2008.

CHALUPKA, A. N.; TALMOR, D. The Economics of sepsis. **Critical Care Clinics**, v. 28, n.1, p. 57-76, Jan., 2012.

COELHO, A.L., HOGABOAM, C.M., KUNKEL, S.L. Chemokines provide the sustained inflammatory bridge between innate and acquired immunity. **Cytokine Growth Factor Reviews**, v.16, n. 6,

p. 553-560, Dec., 2005.

COHEN, J. The immunopathogenesis of sepsis. **Nature**, v. 420, p. 885-91, Dec., 2002.

COIMBRA, R.; SILVERIO, C.C. New mechanical ventilation strategies in acute lung injury and acute respiratory distress syndrome. **Revista de Associação Médica Brasileira**, v. 47, n. 4, p. 358-64, Oct., 2001.

CHANG, HJ; LYNM, C; GLASS, RM. Sepsis. **JAMA**, v. 304, n. 16, p. 1856, Feb., 2010.

CHOPRA, M; JAYNE, S.R; SHARMA, A.C. Acute Lung Injury: Apoptosis and Signaling Mechanisms. **Society for Experimental Biology and Medicine**, v. 234, n. 4, p. 361-371, 2009.

CLARK, S. C. Pulmonary Injury After Extracorporeal Circulation. **Perfusion,** n.2, p. 225-228, 2006.

CUNHA, E.R.; DELARIVA, R.L. Introduction of the bullfrog, *Lithobates catesbeianus* (Shaw, 1802): a review. **Revista Saúde e Biologia,** v. 4, n. 2, p. 34-46, 2009.

CURI, R.; POMPEIA, C.; MIYASAKA, C.K.; PROCOPIO, J. **Understanding fat: fatty acids.** 1 ed., Barueri, SP: Manole, 2002.

DALMORA, M. E. A; DALMORA, S. L.; OLIVEIRA, A. G. Inclusion complex fpiroxican with b-cyclodextrin and incorporation in cationic microemulsions. In vitro drug release and vivo topical anti-inflammatory effect. **International Journal of Pharmaceutics**, v. 222, n. 1, p. 45-55, Jul., 2001.

DAMASCENO, B.P.G.L.; SILVA, J.A.; Oliveira, E.E.; SILVEIRA, W.L.L.; ARAÚJO, I.B.; OLIVEIRA, A.G.; EGITO, E.S.T. Microemulsion: a promising carrier for insoluble molecules. **Revista de Ciências Farmacêuticas Básica e Aplicada,** v. 32, n.1, p. 9-18, 2011.

DELARIVA, R. L.; CUNHA, E. R. Introduction of the bullfrog, Lithobates catesbeianus

(SHAW,1802): a review. **Sabios Revista de Saúde e Biologia**. v. 4, n. 2, p. 34-46, 2009.

DELLINGER, R.P.; LEVY, M.M.; RHODES, A.; ANNANE, D. et.al. Surviving Sepsis Campaign Guidelines Committee Including the Paediatric Subgroup. Surviving Sepsis Campaign: international guidelines for management of severe sepsis and septic shock; **Critical Care Medicine**, v. 41, n. 2, p. 580-637, 2013.

DELLINGER, R.P.; LEVY, M.M.; RHODES, A.; ANNANE, D.; GERLACH, H.; OPAL, S.M.; SEVRANSKY, J.E.; SPRUNG, C.L.; DOUGLAS, I.S.; JAESCHKE, R.; OSBORN, T.M.; NUNNALLY, M.E.; TOWNSEND, S.R.; REINHART, K.; DENNIS, E.A.; NORRIS, P.C. Eicosanoid storm in infection and inflammation. **Nature Reviews Immunology**, v. 15, n. 8, p. 511-523, Aug., 2015.

ELLULU, M.S.; KHAZA'AI, H.; ABED, Y.; RAHMAT, A.; ISMAIL, P.; RANNEH, Y. Role of fish oil in human health and possible mechanism to reduce the inflammation. **Inflammopharmacology**, v. 23, n. 2, p. 79-89, Feb., 2015.

FANTONI, D. T.; AMBROSIO, A.M.; FUTEMA, F.; MIGLIATI, E.R.; TAMURA, E.Y. Use of alfentanil, sufentanil and fentanyl in dogs anaesthetised with halothane. **Ciência Rural**, v.29, n.4, p. 681-688, Oct/Dec, 1999.

FANUN, M. **Microemulsions: Properties and applications**. CRC Taylor & Francis Grourp, Florida, 560p., 2009.

FERRAZ, A.R. Ricardo de Almeida Jorge. Doctor and Humanist from Porto, Timeless Hygienist In - **Arquivos de Medicina**, v. 22, n. 2/3, p. 91-100, 2008.

FIGUEIREDO, K.A.; MENDES, R.M.B.; CARVALHO, A.L.; FREITAS, R.M. Microemulsions for transdermal drug delivery systems: an exploration technology. **Revista GEINTEC**, v.3, n.4, p. 36-46, 2013.

FICETOLA, G.F.; COIC, C.; DETAINT, M.; BERRONEAU, M.; LORVELEC, O.; MIAUD, C. Pettern distribution of the American bullfrog Rana catesbeiana in Europe. **Biological Invasions**, v.9, n.7, p. 767-72, 2007.

FORMARIZ, T. P.; URBAN, M. C. C.; SILVA JÚNIOR, A. A.; GREMIÃO, M. P. D.; OLIVEIRA, A. G. Microemulsion and liquid crystalline phases as drug delivery systems. **Revista Brasileira de Ciências Farmacêuticas**, v. 41, n.3, p. 302-313, 2005.

FUJIHARA M.; MUROI M.; TANAMOTO K.; SUZUKI T.; AZUMA H.; IKEDA H. Molecular mechanisms of macrophage activation and deactivation by lipopolysaccharide: roles of the receptor complex. **Pharmacology & Therapeutics**, v. 100, n. 2, p.171-94, Nov., 2003.

GALLEY H.F.; DUBBELS A.M.; WEBSTER N.R. The effect of midazolam andpropofol on interleukin-8 from human polymorphonuclear leukocytes. **Anesthesia & Analgesia**, v. 86, n. 6, p.1289-93, Jun., 1998.

GILMAN, A.G. **As bases farmacológicas da terapêutica.** 10. ed. Rio de Janeiro: Mcgraw-hill, 2005.

GORDON, L. W.; SHUMMAN, M.; GAO, X.; CHAPMAN, R.; HULDERMAN, T.; SIMEONOVA, P.P. Mechanisms of skeletal muscle injury and repair revealed by gene expression studies in mouse models. **The Journal of Physiology**, v. 582, p. 825-841, Jul., 2007.

GRUPTA, S.; MOULIK, S.P. Biocompatible microemulsions and their prospective uses in drug delivery. **Journal of Pharmaceutical Sciences,** v. 97, n. 1, p. 22-45, Jan., 2008.

HANKE, D.; ZAHRADKA, P.; MOHANKUMAR, S.K.; CLARK, J.L.; TAYLOR, C.G. A diet high in a-linolenic acid and monounsaturated fatty acids attenuates hepatic steatosis and alters hepatic phospholipid fatty acid profile in diet-induced **obese rats.** Prostaglandins, Leukotrienes and Essential Fatty Acids, **v. 89, p. 391-401, Sept., 2013.**

HENKIN, C.S.; COELHO, J.C.; PAGANELLA, M.C.; SIQUEIRA, R.M.; DIAS, F.S. Sepsis: a current view.

Scientia Medica, v. 19, n. 3, p.135-45, jul/set, 2009.

HILÁRIO, M.O.E.; TERRERI, M.T.; LEN, C.A. Non-hormonal anti-inflammatory drugs: cyclooxygenase-2 inhibitors. **Jornal de Pediatria**, v. 82, n. 5, p. 206-212, Nov., 2006.

HOTCHKISS, R.S.; KARL, I.E. The pathophysiology and treatment of sepsis. **The New England Journal of Medicine**, v. 348, p. 138-50, Jan., 2003.

HUBBARD, W.J.; BLAND K.I.; CHAUDRY I.H. The role of the mitochondrion in trauma and shock. **Shock**, v. 22, n. 5, p. 395-402, Nov., 2004.

JADHAV, K.R.; SHETYE, S.L.; KADAM, VJ. Design and Evaluation of Microemulsion Based Drug Delivery System. **International Journal of Advances in Pharmaceutical Sciences**, v.1, p. 156-166, 2010.

JAIMES F. A. Literature review of the epidemiology of sepsis in Latin America. **Revista Panamericana de Salud Publica**, v. 18, n. 3, p. 163-171, 2005.

JOANNE, J.L; GREEN, P.; MANN, J.J.; RAPOPORT, S.I.; SUBLETTE, M.E. Pathways of Polyunsaturated Fatty Acid Utilisation: Implications for Brain Function in Neuropsychiatric Health and Disease. **Brain Research**, v. 9, p. 220246, Feb., 2015.

JOHNSON, K.G.; GHOSE, A.; EPSTEIN, E.; LINCECUM, J.; O'CONNOR, M.B.; VAN VACTOR, D. Axonal heparan sulphate proteoglycans regulate the

distribution and efficiency of the repellent slit during midline axon guidance. **Current Biology**, v. 14, n. 6, p. 499-504, Mar., 2004.

KARIMA, R.; MATSUMOTO, S.; HIGASHI, H.; MATSUSHIMA, K. The molecular pathogenesis of endotoxic shock and organ failure. **Molecular Medicine Today**, v. 5, n. 3, p. 123-132, 1999.

KATZENSTEIN, A.L.A. **Katzenstein and Askin's Surgical Pathology of Non- Neoplastic**

Lung Disease. Major problems in Pathology. 4 ed. Philadephia. PA. Sauders, p. 18-34, 2006.

KAO, S.J.; SU, C.F.; LIU, D.D.; CHEN, H.I. Endotoxin-induced acute lung injury and organ dysfunction are attenuated by pentobarbital anaesthesia. **Clinical and Experimental Pharmacology and Physiology**, v. 34, n. 5-6, p. 480-487, May, 2007.

KAWSKI, C.T.S.; VIEIRA, D.F.V.B.; MOURA JR., D.M.; MADUREIRA, D.S.; ALVES, E.; SILVA, E.S.; GONÇALVES, F.A.F.; GONÇALVES, F.R.; MAIA, F.O.M.; MUSSI, G.M.; DAL SASSO, G.T.M.; ARAÚJO, G.D.G.; LEITE, J.C.R.A.P. **Enfermagem em terapia intensiva: práticas e vivências**. Porto Alegre: Artmed, 2011.

KELBEL, I.; KOCH, T.; WEBER, A.; SCHIEFER, H.G.; VAN ACKERN, K.; NEUHOF, H.; Alterations of bacterial clearance induced by propofol. **Acta Anaesthesiology Scand**, n.43, v. 1, p. 71-76, 1999.

KLEINPELL, R.; AITKEN, L. SCHORR ,C. Implications of the New International Sepsis Guidelines for Nursing Care. **American Journal of Critical Care**, vol. 22 n. 3, p. 212-222. May 2013.

KOENIG, A.; PICON, P.D.; FEIJÓ, J.; SILVA, E.; WESTPHAL, A. Estimation of the economic impact of implementing a hospital protocol for early detection and treatment of severe sepsis in public and private hospitals in southern Brazil. **Revista Brasileira de Terapia Intensiva**, v. 22, n. 3, p. 213-219, Sep., 2010.

KOTANI, N.; HIROSHI, H.; SESSLER, D.I.; TADANOBU, Y.; TOSHIAKI, E.; MASATOSHI, M.; AKITOMO, M. Expression of Genes for Proinflammatory Cytokines in Alveolar Macrophages During Propofol and Isoflurane Anaesthesia. **Anesthesia & Analgesia**, v.89, N. 5, p. 1250-1256, Nov., 1999.

KORTEGEN, A.; HOFMANN, G.; BAUER, M. Sepsis: current aspects of pathophysiology and implications for diagnosis and treatment. **European Journal of Trauma**, v. 32, n. 1, p. 3-9,

Feb., 2006.

KRUMHOLZ, W.; REUSSNER, D.; HEMPELMANN, G. The influence of several intravenous anaesthetics on the chemotaxis of human monocytes in vitro. **European Journal of Anaesthesiology**, v.16, n. 8, p. 547-549, Aug., 1999.

LAGAN, A.L.; MELLEY, D.D.; EVANS, T.W.; QUINILAN, G. J. Pathogenesis of the systemic inflammatory syndrome and acute lung injury: role of iron mobilisation and decompartmentalization. **American Journal of Physiology - Lung Cellular and Molecular Physiology**, n. 294, n. 2, p. 161-174, Feb., 2008.

LEVY, M.M.; FINK, M.P.; MARSHALL, J.C.; ABRAHAM, E.; ANGUS, D; COOK, D. et al. 2001 SCCM/ESICM/ACCP/ATS/SIS International Sepsis Definitions Conference. **Intensive Care Medicine,** v.29, n. 4, p.530-538, April, 2003.

LOBO, S.M.; REZENDE, E.; KNIBEL, M.F.; SILVA, N.B.; PÁRAMO, J.A.M.; NÁCUL, F. et al. Epidemiology and outcome of non-cardiac surgical patients. **Revista Brasileira de Terapia Intensiva**, v. 20, n. 4, p.376-384, Jul., 2008.

LOPES, V.D.S.; DANTAS, T.N.C.; CUNHA, A.F.; MOURA, E.F.; MACIEL, A.M. Obtaining an anionic surfactant from *Rana Catesbeiana* SHAW oil. **Revista de Ciência e Vida,** v.30, n.2, p.85-97, jul-dez 2010.

LOPES, V.D.S. **Bullfrog oil: A physical-chemical study aimed at pharmacological activity.** Dissertation (Master's Degree) Department of Chemistry, Federal University of Rio Grande do Norte, 2007.

LUCAS, S. The autopsy pathology of sepsis-related death. **Current Diagnostic Pathology**, vol. 13, N. 5, p.375-388, Oct., 2007.

LYONS, C. L., E. B. KENNEDY; ROCHE, H.M. Metabolic Inflammation- Differential Modulation by

Dietary Constituents. **Nutrients**, v. 8, n. 5, p. 247, April, 2016.

MACEDO-NETO, A.V.; SANTOS, L.V.; MENEZES, S.L.; PAIVA, D.S.; ROCCO, P.R.; ZIN, W.A. Respiratory mechanics after prosthetic reconstruction of the chest wall in normal rats. **Chest**, v. 113, n. 6, p.1667-72, Jun., 1998.

MAKSYMCHUK, O.V. The influence of omega-3 polyunsaturated fatty acids on the expression of enzymes of the prooxidant and antioxidant systems in the rat liver. **Fiziolohichnyi Zhurnal**, v. 60, n. 3, p. 32-37, 2014.

MARSHALL, J. C.; PANACEK, E. A.; Teoh, L. et al. Modelling organ dysfunction as a risk factor, outcome, and measure of biologic effect in sepsis. **Critical Care Medicine,** v. 28: A46, 2001.

MARTIN, G.S.; MANNINO, D.M.; EATON S. et al; The epidemiology of sepsis in the United States from 1979 through 2000. **New England Journal of Medicine**, v. 348, p.1546-1554, 2003.

MARTINS, M.B.; SUAIDEN, A.S.; PIOTTO, R.F.; BARBOSA, M. Properties of polyunsaturated fatty acids - Omega 3 obtained from fish oil and linseed oil. **Revista do Instituto de Ciências da Saúde**, v. 26, n. 2, p. 153156, 2008.

McGILL, S.N.; AHMED, N.A.; CHRISTOU, N.V. Endothelial cell: role in infection and inflammation. **World Journal of Surgical,** v.22, p.171-178, 1998.

MEDZHITOV, R.; JANEWAY JR., C.A. Innate immune recognition and control of adaptive immune responses. **Seminars in Immunology,** v. 10, n. 5, p. 3513, Oct., 1998.

MÉNDEZ, E.; SANHUEZA, J.; NIETO, S.; SPEISKY, H.; VENENZUELA, A. Fatty acid composition, extraction, fractionation and stabilisation of bullfrog (Rana catesbeiana) oil. Journal of the American Oil Chemists' Society, v.75, n.1, p.79-83, Jan., 1998.

MILLER, W. C.; SWYGARD, H.; HOBBS, M. M.; FORD, C. A.; HANDCOCK, M. S.; MORRIS, M.; SCHMITZ, J. L.; COHEN, M. S.; HARRIS, K. M.; UDRY, J. R. The prevalence of trichomoniasis in young adults in the United States. **Journal of the American Sexually Transmitted Diseases**, v. 32, n. 10, p. 593-598, Oct., 2005.

MILIC, S.; LULIC, D.; STIMAC, D. Non-alcoholic fatty liver disease and obesity: Biochemical, metabolic and clinical presentations. **World Journal of Gastroenterology**, v. 20, n. 28, p. 9330-9337, Jul. 2014.

MOUTA JUNIOR, MF. **Increased survival and decreased expression of actin and fibronectin in the thymus, in sepsis treated with thymus explant supernatant.** Dissertation (Master's Degree), Faculty of Medicine, University of São Paulo, 2007.

MONTEIRO et al. Ultra-processing and a new classification of foods. In: NEEF. R. (Ed). **Introduction to U.S. Food System: Public Health, Environment, and Equity**. San Francisco: Jossey-Bass A Wiley Brand, 2014.

MUZAFFAR, F.; SINGH, U. K.; CHAUHAN, L. Review on microemulsion as futuristic drug delivery. **International Journal of Pharmacy Pharmaceutical Sciences**, v.5, n.3, p.39-53, 2013.

NAJJAR, R. **Microemulsions: An Introduction to Properties and Applications**. Croatia: Intech, 2012.

NÓBREGA, I.C.C.; ATAÍDE, C.S.; MOURA, O.M.; LIVERA, A.V; MENEZES, P.H. Volatile constituents of cooked bullfrog (Rana catesbeiana) legs. **Food Chemistry**, v.102, n.1, p.186-191, 2007.

NASCIUTTI, P.R.; COSTA, A.P.A.C.; SANTOS JÚNIOR, M.B.; MELO, N.G.; CARVALHO, R.O.A. Fatty acids and the cardiovascular system. Enciclopédia biosfera. **Centro Científico Conhecer**, v.11, n.22; p.11-29, Dec., 2015.

O'BRIEN, J.M.; NAEEM, A.A.; ABEREGG, S.K.; ABRAHAM, E. Sepsis. The American Journal of Medicine, v. 120, p. 1012-22, Dec., 2007.

PARKER, J.C; GILLESPIE, M.N.; TAYLOR, A.E.; MARTIN, S.L. Capillary filtration coefficient, vascular resistance, and compliance in isolated mouse lungs. **Journal of Applied Physiology**, v. 87, n. 4, p.1421-7, Oct.,1999.

PASCOA, H.; DINIZ, D.G.A.; FLORENTINO, I.F.; COSTA, E.A.; BARA, M.T.F. Microemulsion based on Pterodon emarginatus oil and its anti-inflammatory potential. **Brazilian Journal of Pharmaceutical Sciences**, v. 51, n. 1, p. 117126, Jan./Mar., 2015.

PESCE, C.; DELGADO, S.M. Ácidos grasos omega 3: respuesta inmune y su efecto sobre algunas enfermedades. **Enfermería**, v. 3, n. 1, p. 33-37, Jun., 2014.
PEREIRA, B. Oxygen free radicals and their importance for immunological functionality. **Motriz**, v.2, n.2, Dec., 1996.

PEREZ M.C.A. **Epidemiology, diagnosis, immunocompetence markers and prognosis of sepsis.** Thesis (Doctorate) - School of Medical Sciences, Rio de Janeiro State University, 2009.

PERINI, J. A. L.; STEVANATO, F. B.; SARGI, S. C.; VISENTAINER, J. E. L.; DALALIO, M. M. O.; MATSHUSHITA, M.; SOUZA, N. E.; VISENTAINER, J. V. Polyunsaturated fatty acids n-3 and n-6: metabolism in mammals and immune response. **Revista de Nutrição**, v, 23, n. 6, p. 1075-1086, Nov./Dec., 2010.

PEREIRA, M. M. **Growth and nutrient deposition of bullfrogs during fattening: adjustment of non-linear models.** Thesis (PhD) - Paulista State University, Aquaculture Centre, 2013.

PETÁK, F.; HABRE, W.; HANTOS, Z.; SLY, P.D.; MOREL, D.R. Effects of pulmonary vascular pressures and flow on airway and parenchymal mechanics in isolated rat lungs. **Journal of Applied Physiology**, v. 92, n. 1, p. 169-78, Jan., 2002.

POLETTO, A. C. **Unsaturated fatty acids oleic and linoleic repress the Slc2a4 gene via NF-kB and SRPB1.** Thesis (PhD) - University of São Paulo. São Paulo, 2011.

POLYZOS, S.A.; KOUNTOURAS, J.; ZAYOS, C.; DERETZI, G. The Association Between Helicobacter pylori Infection and Insulin Resistance: A Systematic Review. **Helicobacter**, v. 16, n.2, p. 79-88, April, 2011.

PROULX, F.; FAYON, M.; FARRELL, C.A.; LACROIX, J.; GAUTHIER, M. Epidemiology of sepsis and multiple organ dysfunction syndrome in children. **Chest**, v.109, p.1033-1037, April, 1996.

RABAUEL, C.; MEBAZAA, A. Septic shock: a heart story since the 1960s. **Intensive Care Medicine**, v. 32, n. 6, p. 799-807, Jun., 2006.

RAMOS, A.C.S. **Tungsten extraction using microemulsions.** Dissertation (Master's Degree) - Technology Centre, Chemical Engineering Department, Postgraduate Programme in Chemical Engineering, Federal University of Rio Grande do Norte, Natal, 1996.

REVERÓN, F F. Acute pulmonary injury. **Revista Cubana Medicina Militar**, v.29, n.2, p.118-126, 2000.

ROBBINS, S.L.; COTRAN, R. S.; KUMAR, V. Robbins: **Structural and Functional Pathology.** 6. ed. Rio de Janeiro: Granabara Koogan, 2000.

ROSSI, C. G. F. T.; DANTAS, T. N. C. ; NETO, A. A. D. ; MACIEL, M. A. M. Microemulsions: a basic approach and prospects for applicability

industrial. **Revista Universitária Rural. Exact and Earth Sciences Series, Seropédica,** vol. 26, n. 1-2, p. 45-66, Jan/Dec, 2007.

RUTH M.; ANGUS, D.C.; DEUTSCHMAN, C.S.; MACHADO, F.R.; RUBENFELD, G.D.; WEBB, S.A.; BEALE, R.J.; VINCENT, J.; MORENO, R. Surviving Sepsis Campaign: International guidelines for the treatment of severe sepsis and septic shock: 2012. **Critical Care Medicine**, v. 41, n. 2, 2013.

RUSSEL, J.A. Management of sepsis. **The New England Journal of Medicine**, v. 355, p. 1699-713, Oct., 2006.

SALES JÚNIOR, J.A.; DAVID, C.M.; HATUM, R. Sepsis Brazil: epidemiological study of sepsis in Brazilian intensive care units. **Revista Brasileira de Terapia Intensiva**, v.18, n. 1, p.18-19, Jan/Mar., 2006.

SCORLETTI, E.; BYRNE, C.D. Omega-3 Fatty Acids, Hepatic Lipid Metabolism, and Nonalcoholic Fatty Liver Disease. **Annual Review of Nutrition**. v.33. p. 231-48, Jul., 2013.

SHAKEEL, F.; RAMADAN, W. Transdermal delivery of anticancer drug caffeine from water-in-oil nanoemulsions. **Colloids and Surface B: Biointerfaces**, v.75, n. 1, p.356-362, Sep., 2010.

SILVA, E.; PEDRO, M.A.; SOGAYAR, A.C.; MOHOVIC, T.; SILVA, C.L.; JANISZEWSKI M.; CAL, R.G.; DE SOUSA, E.F.; ABE, T.P.; ANDRADE, J.; MATOS, J.D.; REZENDE, E.ASSUNÇÃO, M.; AVEZUM, A.; ROCHA P.C.; MATOS, G.F.; BENTO, A.M.; CORRÊA, A.D.; VIEIRA, P.C.; KNOBEL, E. Brazilian Sepsis Epidemiological Study. **Critical Care**, v.8, n.4, p.251-260, August, 2004.

SILVA, J.A.; SANTANA, D.P.; BEDOR, D.C.G.; BORBA, V.F.C.; LIRA, A.A.M.; EGITO, E.S.T. In vitro release and permeation study of diclofenac diethylammonium in gel-like microemulsion. **Química Nova**, v.32, n.6, p. 1389-1393, Jul., 2009.

SILVA, P.L.; ABREU M.G. How to Determine Volemia in Patients with Acute Lung Injury/Acute Respiratory Distress Syndrome. **Sumário Content Editorial**, v. 20, n. 1, p. 4742, 2011.

SIQUEIRA-BATISTA, R.; GOMES, A.P.; PESSOA-JÚNIOR, V.P. Sepsis: updates and perspectives. **Revista Brasileira de Terapia Intensiva**, v. 23, n. - 2, p. 207-216, April/June, 2009.

SOUSA, A.W.P; ARAÚJO, M.S.T; HENRIQUES, M.S.M. Pathophysiological mechanisms involved in the development of non-alcoholic steatohepatitis. **Medicina & Pesquisa**, v. 1, n. 1, Jan./April, 2015.

SZOSTAK, A.; **OGtUSZKA,** M.; PAS, M.F.W.T; **POtAWSKA,** E.; URBANSKI, P.; USZCZUK-KUBIAK, E.; BLICHARSKI, T.; CHANDRA, S.P.; DUNKELBERGER, J.R.;

HORBANCZUK, J.O.; **PIERZCHALA,** A. Effect of a diet enriched with omega-6 and omega-3 fatty acids on the pig liver transcriptome. **Genes & Nutrition**, v. 11, n. 9, Mar., 2016.

TANIGUCHI, T.; SHIBATA, K.; YAMAMOTO, K. Ketamine inhibits endotoxininduced shock in rats. **Anesthesiology**, v. 95, n. 4, p. 928-932, Oct., 2001.

THAN, N.N.; NEWSOME, P.N. A concise review of non-alcoholic fatty liver disease. **Atherosclerosis**, v. 239, n. 1, p. 192-202, Mar., 2015.

THOMAS, M.S.; MITCHELL, J. S.; DENUCCI, C.C.; MARTIN, A.L.; SHIMIZU, 7
Y. The p110 isoform of phosphatidylinositol 3-kinase regulates migration of effector CD4 T lymphocytes into peripheral inflammatory sites. **Journal of Leukocyte Biology**, v. 84, n.3, p.814-823, Jun., 2008.

TSOCHATZIS, E.A.; PAPATHEODORIDIS, G.V.; ARCHIMANDRITIS, A.J. Adipokines in nonalcoholic steatohepatitis: from pathogenesis to implications in diagnosis and therapy. **Mediators of inflammation**, April, 2009.

ÚSTÚNDAÕ OKUR, N.; APAYDIN, S.; YAVAÇOÕLU, N. U. K.; YAVAÇOÕLU, A.; KARASULU, H. Y. Evaluation of skin permeation and anti-inflammatory and analgesic effects of new naproxen microemulsion formulations. **International Journal of Pharmaceutics**, v. 416, n. 1, p. 136-144, Sep., 2011.

VIANA, R. A. P. P.; WHITAKER, I. Y.; ALBUQUERQUE, A.M.; BALSANELLI, A.P.; QUEIJO, A.F.; PIETRO, A.; SILVA, A.B.V.; YOSHITOME, A.Y.; BEZERRA, A.L.; MESQUITA, A.; ARÃO, B.T.F.; CARNEIRO, C.S.; BRITO, C.M.; CAIXETA, C.R.; FARIAS, C.; MARCELINO, C.A.G.; COHRS, C.R.; MATSUBA, C.S.T.; VINCENT, J.L.; BIHARI D.J.; SUTER, P.M.; BRUINING, H.A.; WHITE, J.; NICOLAS-CHANOIN M.H. The prevalence of nosocomial infection in intensive care units in Europe. Results of the European Prevalence of Infection in Intensive Care (EPIC) Study. In: EPIC International Advisory Committee. **JAMA**, v.274, n.8, p.639-644, Aug., 1995.

VINCENT, J.L.; SAKR, Y.; SPRUNG, C.; RANIERI, V.; REINHART, K.; GERLACH, H.; MORENO R.; CARLET J.; LE GALL J.R.; PAYEN D. Sepsis in European intensive care units: results of the SOAP study. **Critical Care of Medicine**, v. 34, n. 2, p. 344-353, Feb., 2006.

WARE L. B. Pathophysiology of acute lung injury and the acute respiratory distress syndrome. **Seminars in Respiratory and Critical Care Medicine**, v. 27, n.4, p. 337-49, Aug., 2006.

WHEELLER, A.P.; BERNARD, G.R. Treating patients with severe sepsis. **The New England Jounal of Medicine**, v. 340, n. 3, p. 207-214, Jan., 1999.

WINSOR, P. A. Hydrotopy, solubilisation and related emulsification processes I to VIII. **Transaction Faraday Society** , v.44, 376-398, 1948.

YURDAKOC, A.; GUNDAY, I.; MEMIS, D. Effects of halothane, isoflurane, and sevoflurane on lipid peroxidation following experimental closed head trauma in rats. **Acta Anaesthesiologica Scandinava**, v. 52, n. 5, p. 658-663, May, 2008.

XIE, X.; RIVIER, A.; ZAKRZEWICZ, A.; BERNIMOULIN, M.; ZENG, X.; WESSEL, H.P.; SCHAPIRA, M.; SPERTINI, O. Inhibition of Selectin-mediated Cell Adhesion and Prevention of Acute Inflammation by Nonanticoagulant Sulfated. **The Journal of Biological Chemistry**, v. 275, n. 44, p. 34818-34825, Nov., 2000.

XIER, X.; RIVIER, A.S.; ZAKRZEWICZ, A.; BERNIMOULIN, M.; ZENG X.L.; WESSEL, H.P.; SCHPIRA, M.; SPERTINI, O. Inhibition of selectin-mediated cell adhesion and prevention of acute inflammation by nonanticoagulant sulfated saccharides. Studies with carboxyl-reduced and sulfated heparin and with trestatin a sulfate. **Journal of Biology Chemistry**, v.275, n.44, p.34818-34825, Nov., 2000.

ZANON, F.; JAIRO, C. Sepsis in the intensive care unit: etiologies, prognostic factors and mortality. **Revista Brasileira de Terapia Intensiva**, v.20, n.2, p. 128-134, April/June, 2008.

ZUG, G.R.; VITT, L.J.; CALDWELL, J.P. **Herpetology: An Introductory Biology of Amphibians and Reptiles**. San Diego - California - USA: Academic Press, 2 ed., 2001.

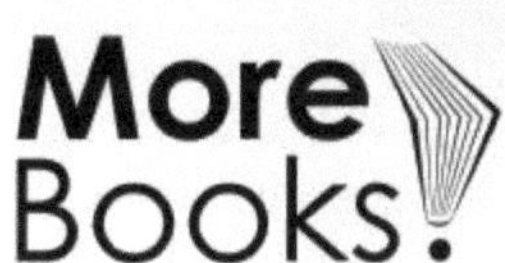

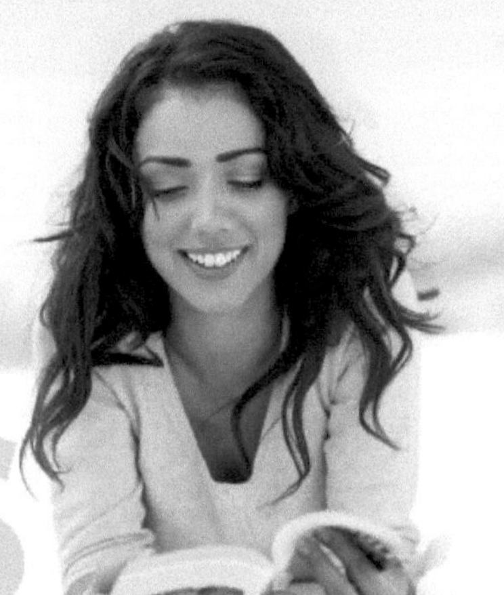

yes

I want morebooks!

Buy your books fast and straightforward online - at one of world's fastest growing online book stores! Environmentally sound due to Print-on-Demand technologies.

Buy your books online at
www.morebooks.shop

Kaufen Sie Ihre Bücher schnell und unkompliziert online – auf einer der am schnellsten wachsenden Buchhandelsplattformen weltweit! Dank Print-On-Demand umwelt- und ressourcenschonend produzi ert.

Bücher schneller online kaufen
www.morebooks.shop

info@omniscriptum.com
www.omniscriptum.com

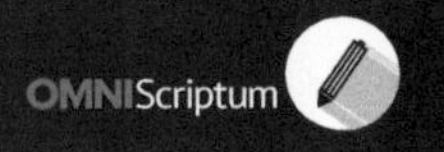

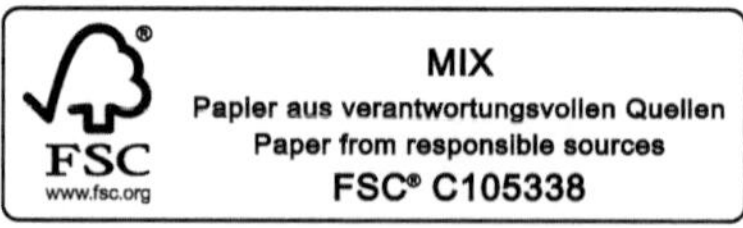

Printed by Books on Demand GmbH, Norderstedt / Germany